PATCH LAND ADVENTURES

BOOK THREE

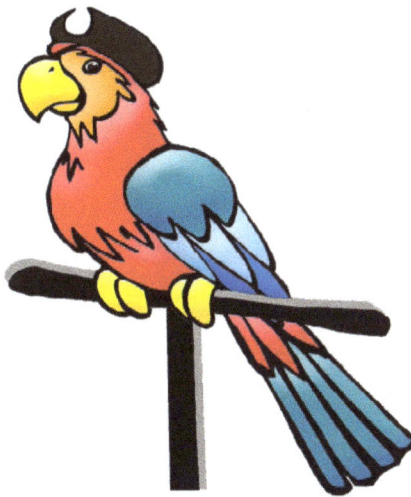

PIRATE'S ADVENTURE

WRITTEN BY CARMEN SWICK
ILLUSTRATED BY JOEY MANFRE

For information go to: www.presbeaupublishing.com or email carmens222@gmail.com

The author of this book does not dispense medical advice or prescribe the use of any technique as a form of treatment physical or emotional, or medical problems without the advice of a physician, either directly or indirectly. The intent of the author is to share her story about her son and to help those with eye patching to be able to use this book as a tool, and for the children that do not need to eye patch, they will enjoy the fiction adventures the story delivers.

Carmen Swick's Editor: Page Lambert
Illustrator: Joey Manfre
Cover design by: Joey Manfre
Carmen Swick's Head Shot by: MDphotonet.com

PRESBEAU
PUBLISHING

Publisher: Presbeau Publishing Inc.
ISBN# 978-0-9831380-2-0
Library of Congress Control Number: 2013917665

Printed and Bound and Published in the United States of America

Patch Land Adventures: Pirate's Adventure www.patchlandadventures.com

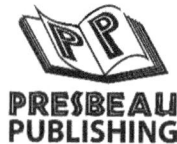

FOREWARD

Carmen has written yet another powerful, fun-filled book about Patch Land Adventures! Pirate's Adventure is more than a story about children facing challenges. It is a story about friendship, family, pets, and community, and how these can work together to provide support and a foundation for our children. It's a book about strength, encouragement, as well as about children and parents developing abilities to overcome or manage personal challenges by sometimes learning to turn them into adventures. Each of us has challenges; it's just that for some, they are more visible than for others. Bravo for Patch Land Adventures!

David A. Dixon - Author of *Notes to My Daughter* and *Notes to My Son.*

Pirate's Adventure is a fun-filled book that shows the importance of friendship, having fun, and being there for those you care about, in good times and tough times. I love that the Patch Land Adventures books normalize patching and eye exams for kids, and show them that adventures can happen to anyone. Book 3: Pirate's Adventure definitely shows that there's really nothing that keeps kids from a good adventure.

Ann Zawistoski, Author of *Glasses: a board book* and owner of the Little Four Eyes website.

No one wants to be different. We grow up simply wanting to fit in. Through Carmen's book series, Patch Land Adventures, she speaks to the kid in all of us. She tells us it's alright to be distinct and encourages us to be accepting. Every one of us needs to live with the truth that we are all just "patching" our way through life—and that we can do anything.

Dawna Hetzler, Award-winning author of *Walls of a Warrior*, Speaker.

DEDICATIONS AND ACKNOWLEDGMENTS

Dedicated to Beau
January 8, 2002- June 12, 2015

This book is dedicated to my son Preston who truly inspired me to write Patch Land Adventures book and turn it into a series. Patching did not stop Preston from doing what he loves! Preston's diligence in patching to help improve his eyesight was outstanding. He was committed to the efforts required and pushed ahead through the tough times and set-backs. I love you and thank you for not giving up.

Special thanks, to my family and friends for their support and believing I could write our story to share with many. Mimi thank you for always being so supportive and creative with all the incentive packages you sent Preston to stay on course.

Page Lambert, my editor, you were so kind and patient with me and not only helped with the editing, you also guided me through the process.

Joey Manfre, my illustrator, thank you for bringing Patch Land Adventures series Book One: "Fishing with Grandpa", Book Two: "Camping at Mimi's Ranch", and Book Three: "Pirates Adventure" to life with your illustrations and being my my creative partner, to help tell the story through the author's vision! Your gift as an artist truly shows through your work. I am happy to say that I have also found a friend.

Let's not forget our dog Beau who is a Weimaraner, Preston's eye patch buddy in the Patch Land Adventures. Beau has a very special bond with Preston.

"Beau, today is a special day.
It is my birthday. I am having a pirate's party.
Tommy, Billy and Missy and the rest
of my friends and family are coming over."

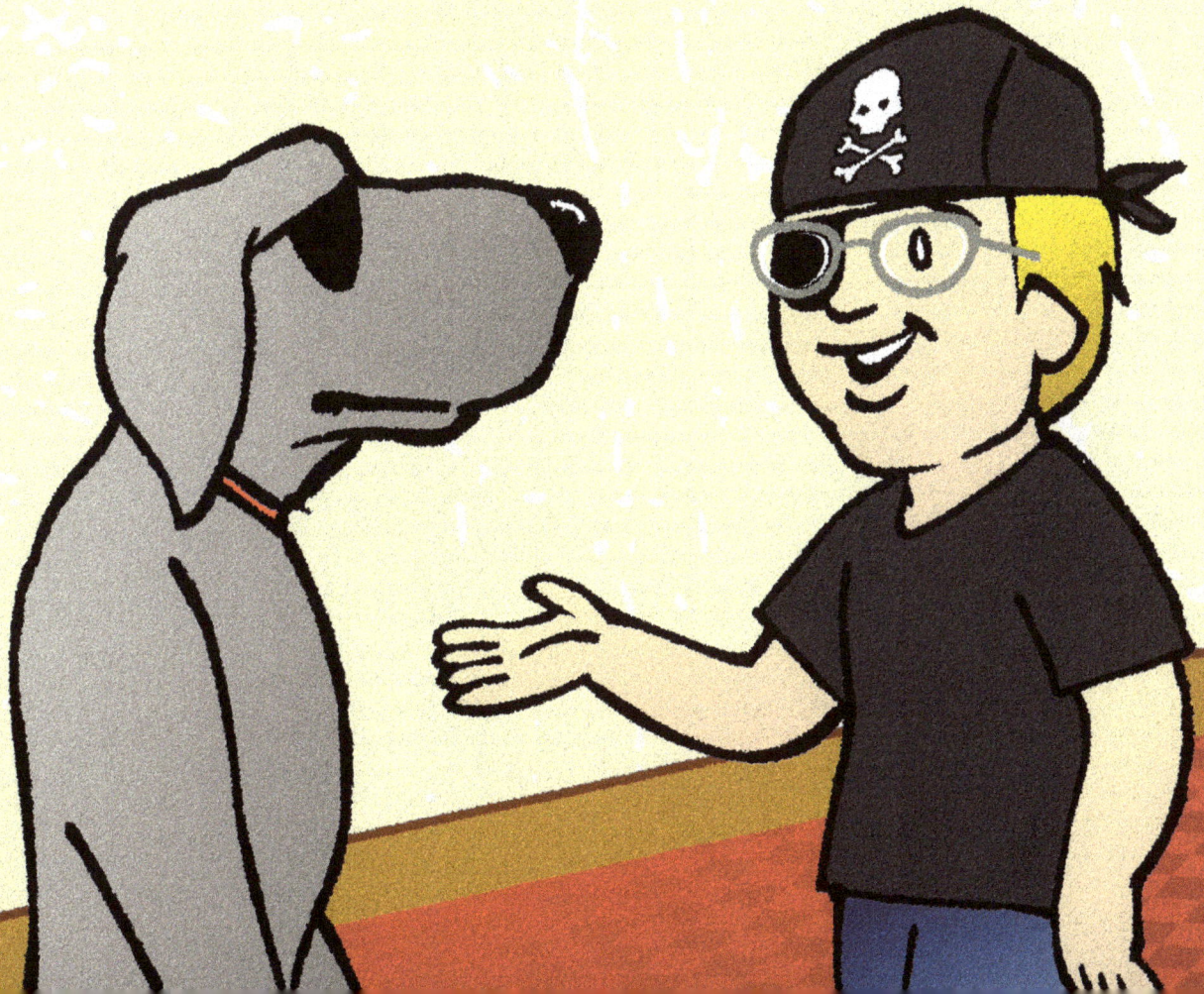

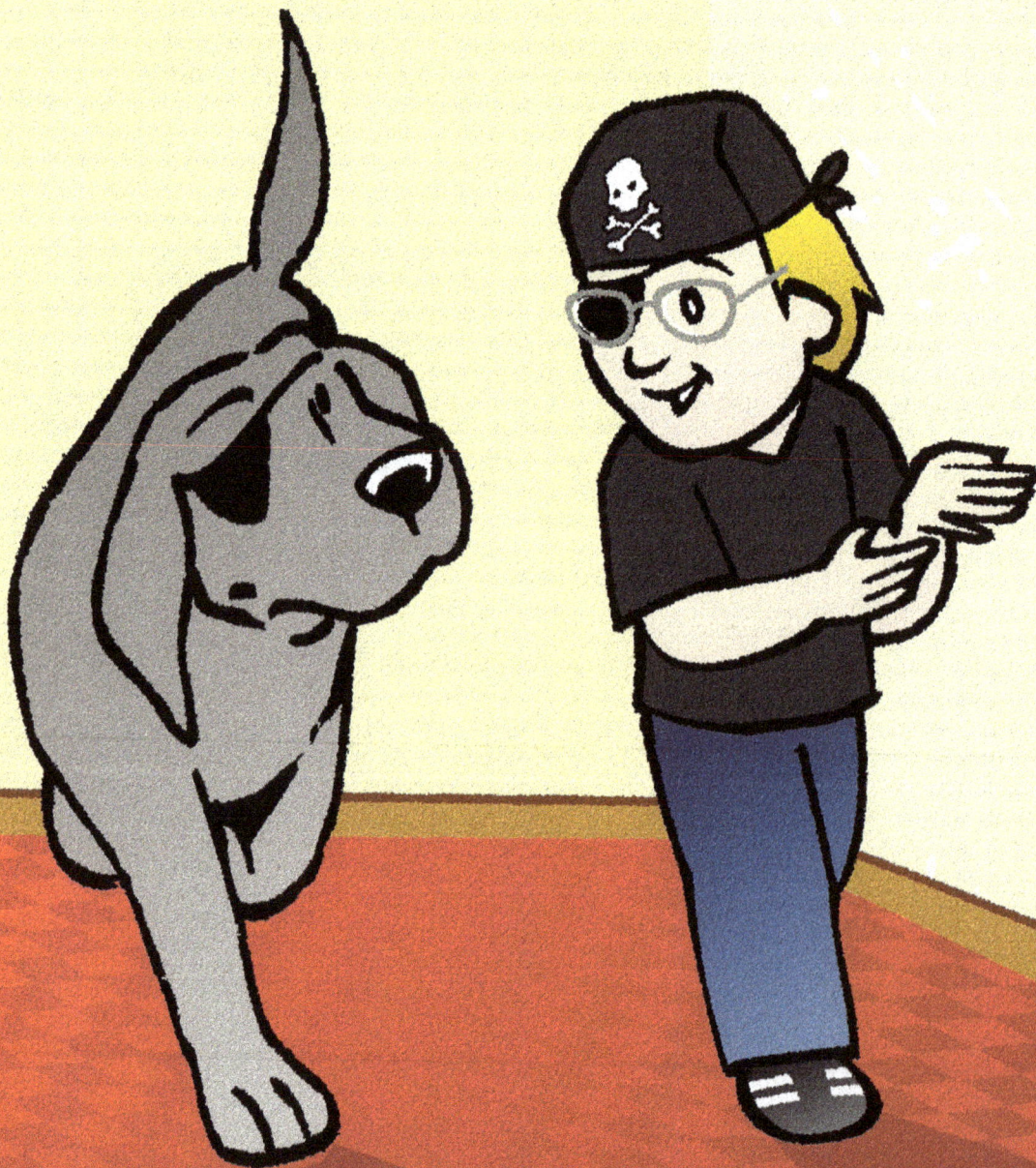

"I am so excited. Mom made me a cake that looks like a treasure chest. "My piñata looks like a treasure chest too."

"Since it is a pirate's party, everyone will be wearing a pirate's patch. Grandpa, do you think my friends will wear their pirates' patches for my birthday party?"

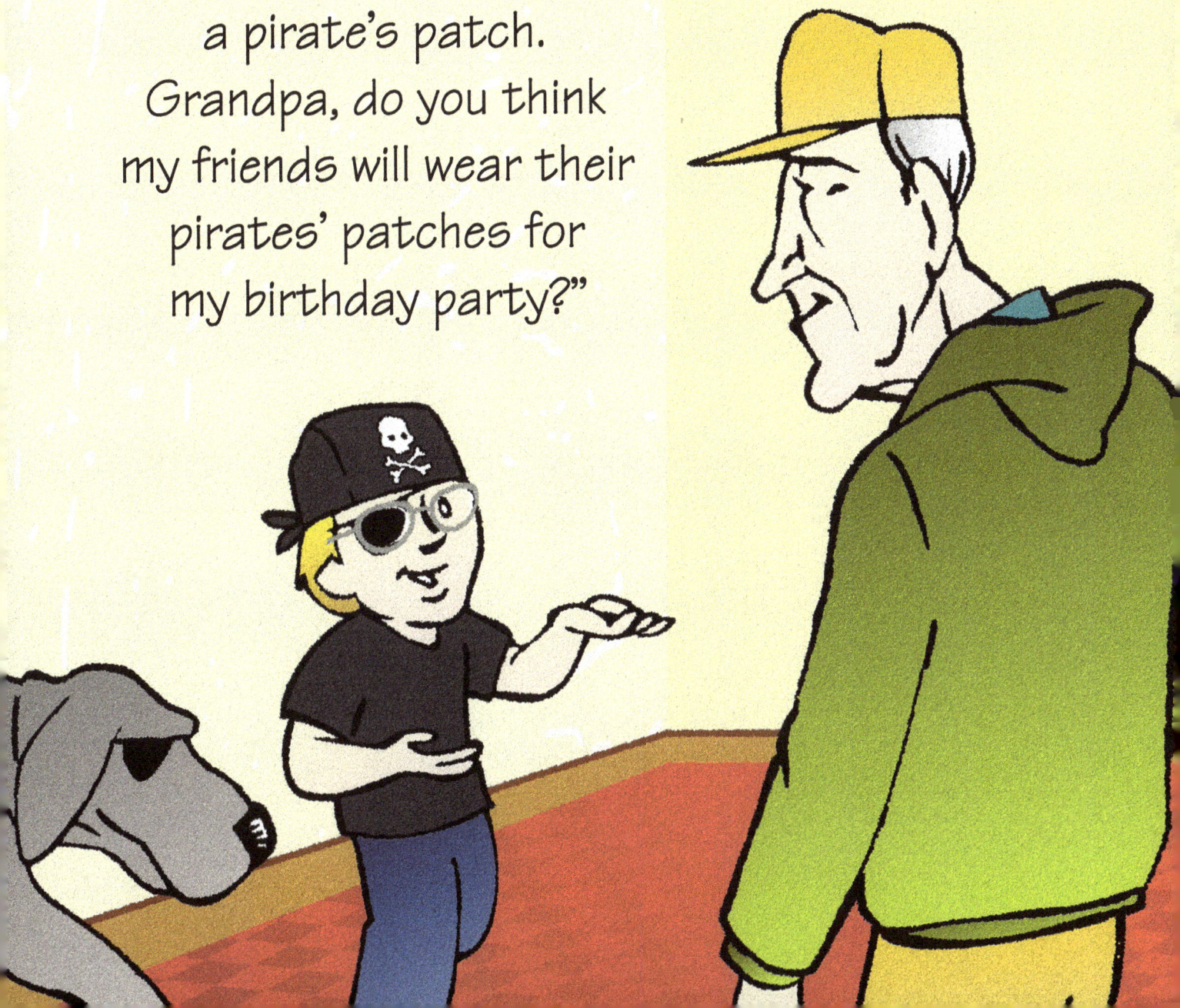

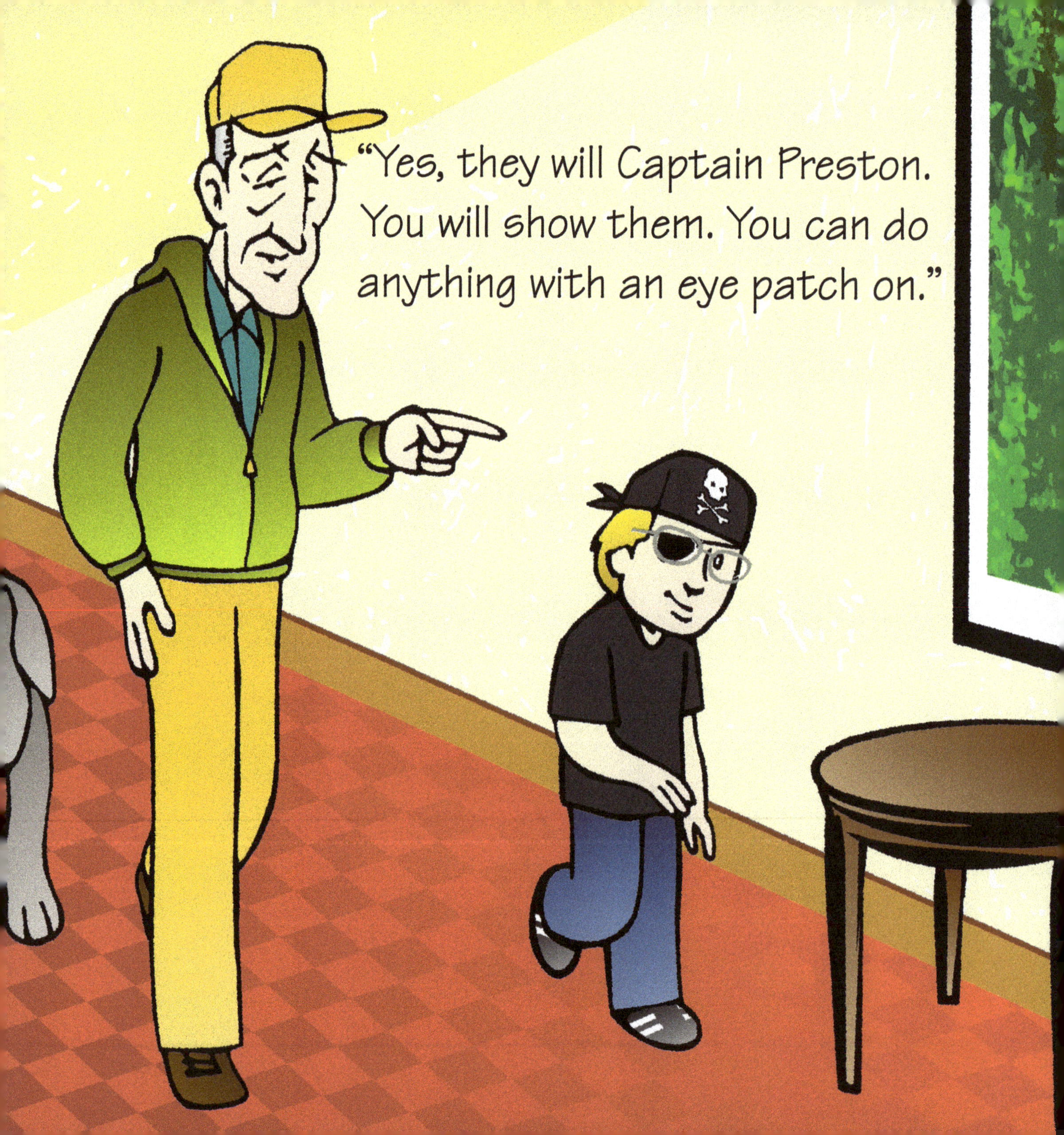
"Yes, they will Captain Preston. You will show them. You can do anything with an eye patch on."

"Mom, Dad, all of my
friends and cousins are here!
Let's all go down to
the basement."

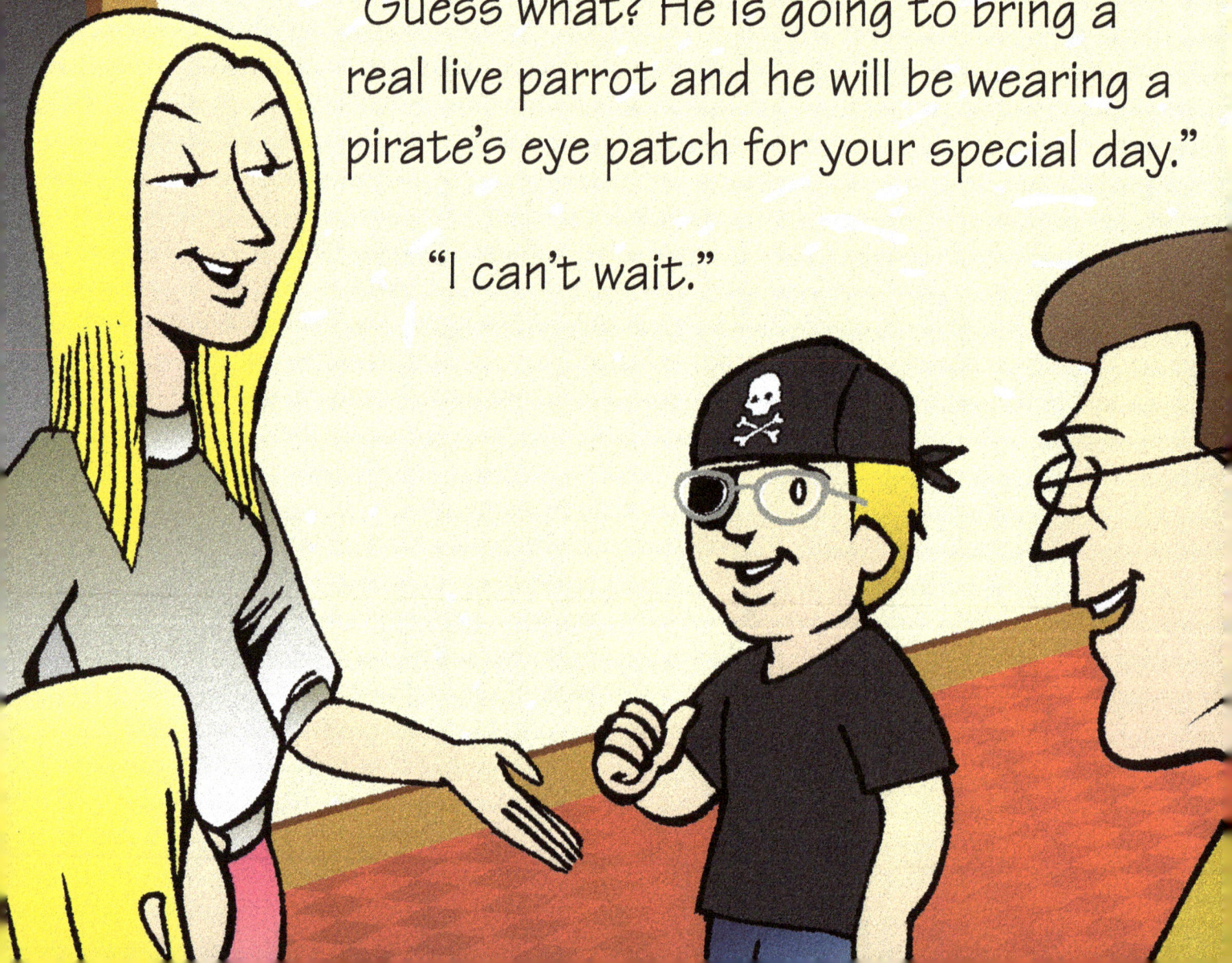

"Wait, Preston. Dad and I want to tell you that Coco the Pirate Clown is coming over as a surprise."

"Guess what? He is going to bring a real live parrot and he will be wearing a pirate's eye patch for your special day."

"I can't wait."

"Ahoy, mates, let's hit the piñata for the pirate's treasure."

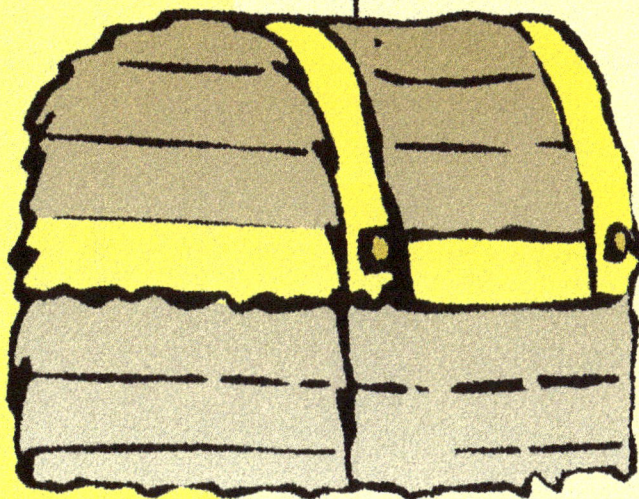

"I get to hit it first because it is my birthday."

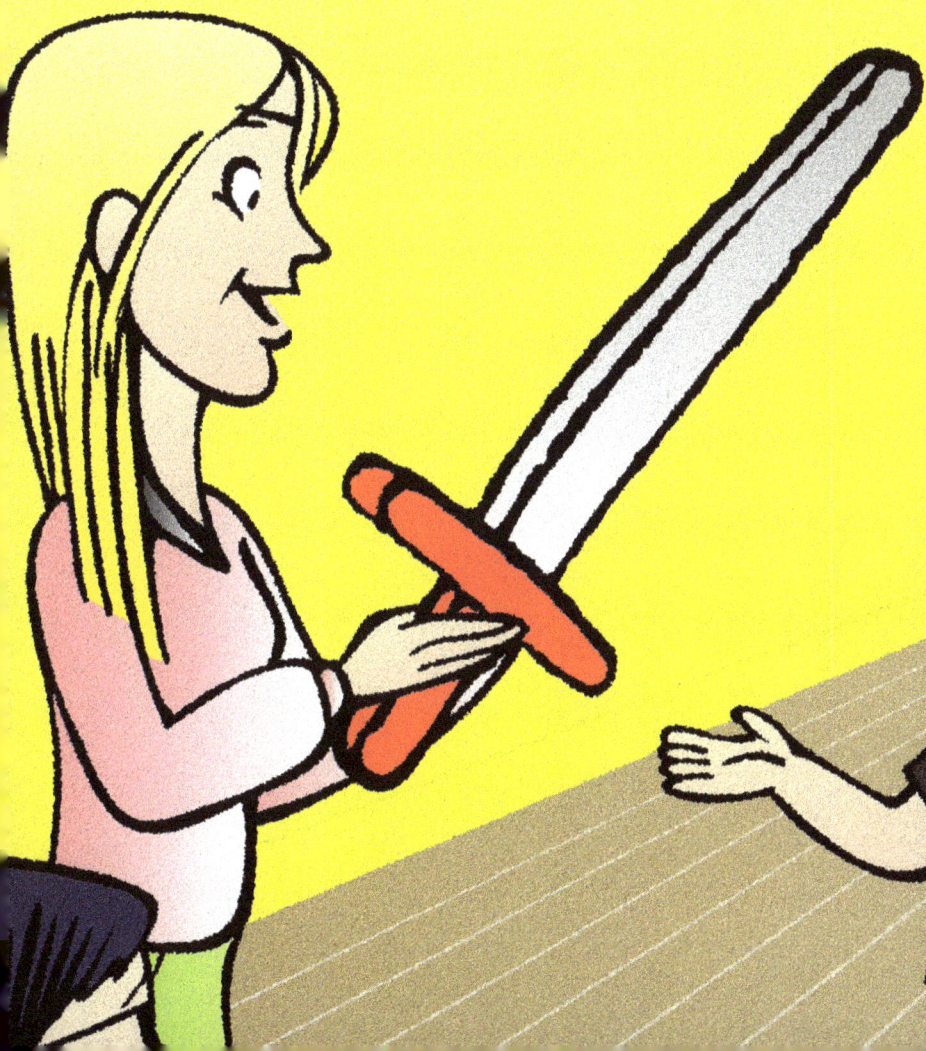

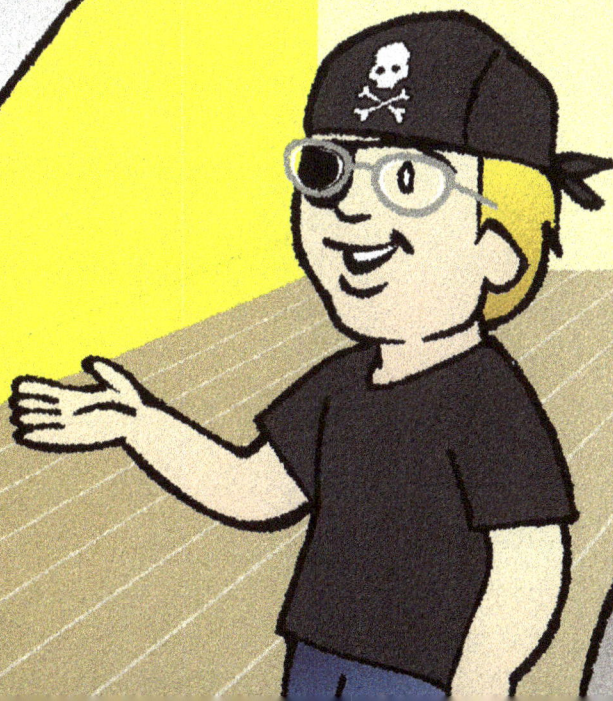

"Preston, it will be too hard to hit the piñata with a patch on."

"No, it's not Billy Watch me! We can do anything with an eye patch on. Right, Tommy?"

"You bet, Captain Preston!"

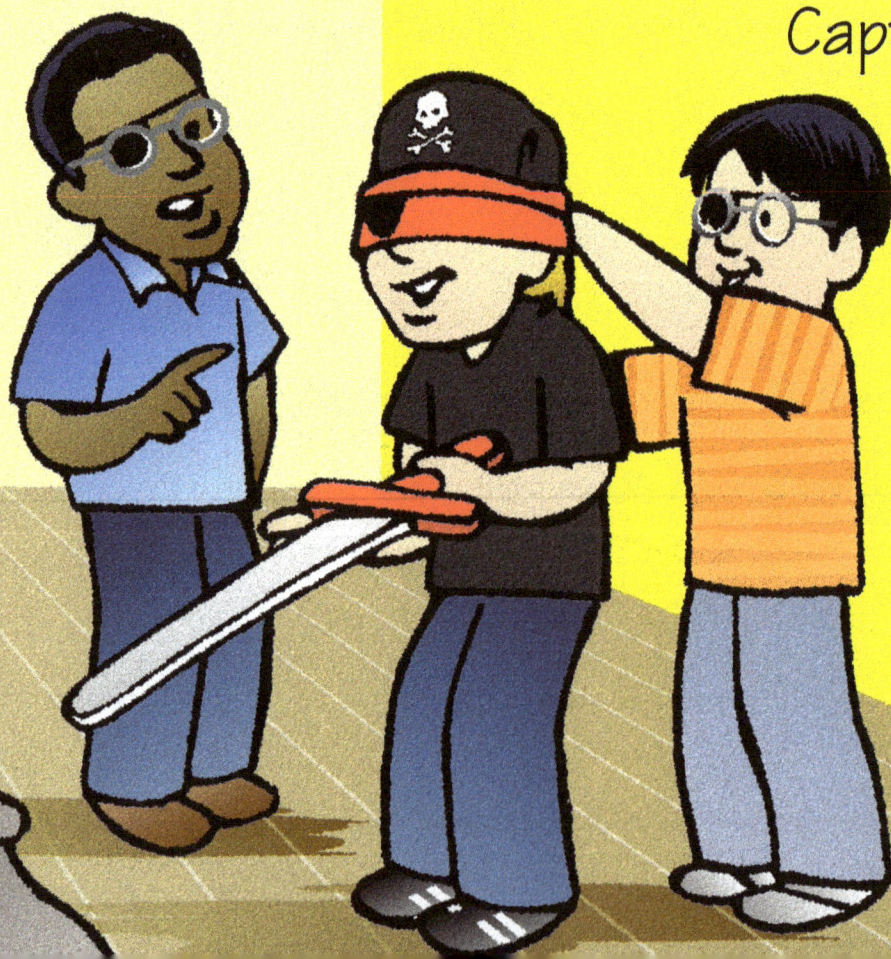

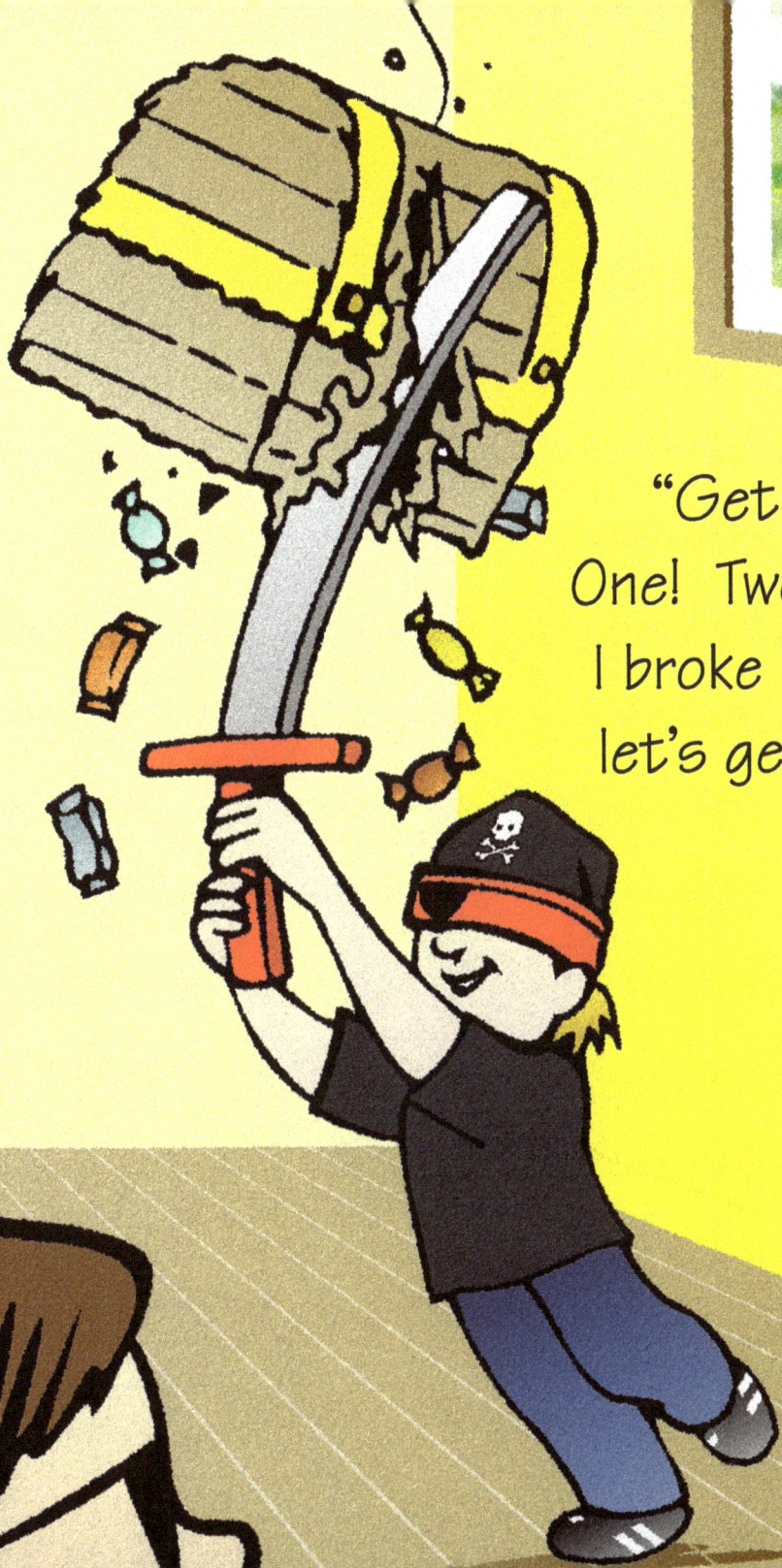

"Get back, mates.
One! Two! Three! Bang!!
I broke it! Argh, mates,
let's get the treasure."

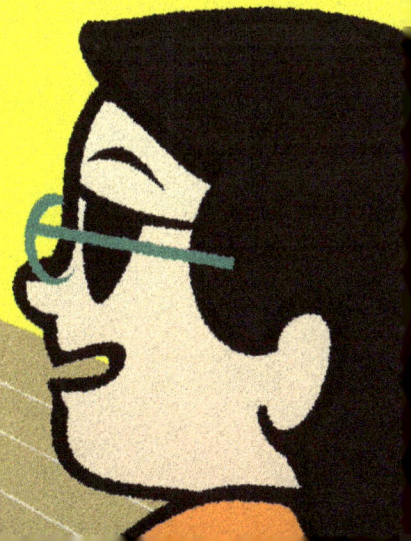

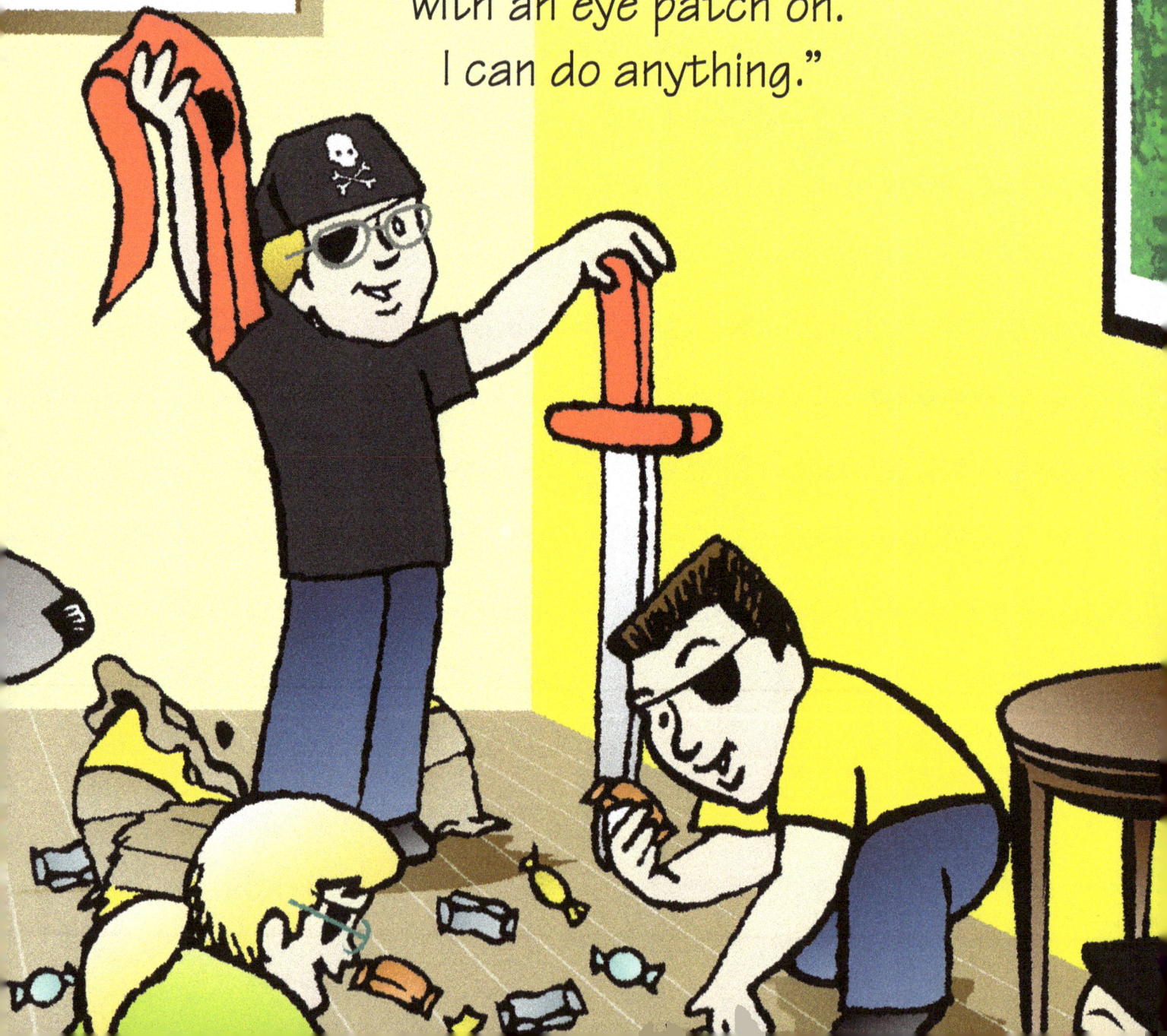

"Shipmates, I did it with an eye patch on. I can do anything."

"Ahoy, mates. I am Coco the Pirate Clown, here to see Captain Preston for his birthday."

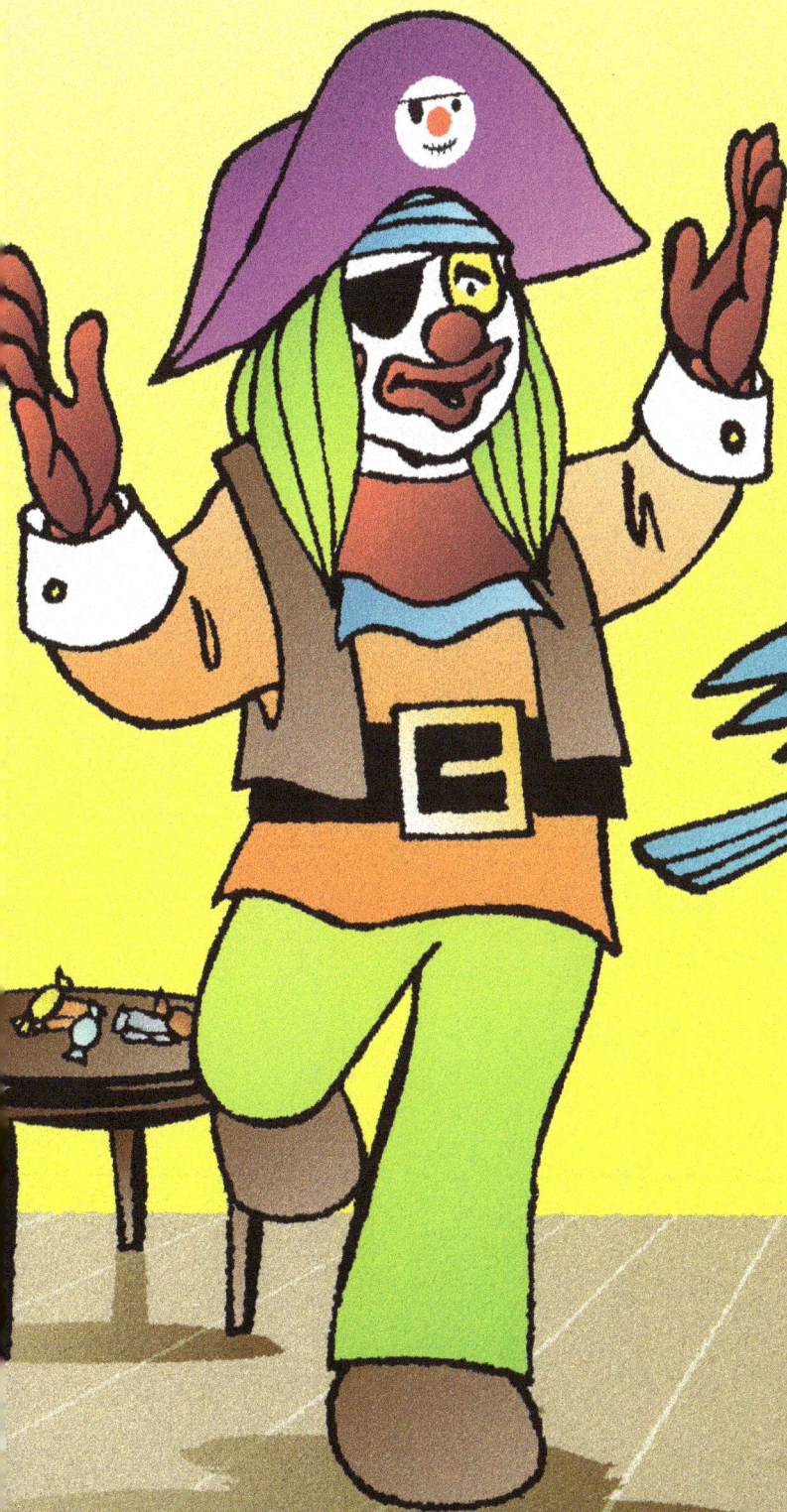

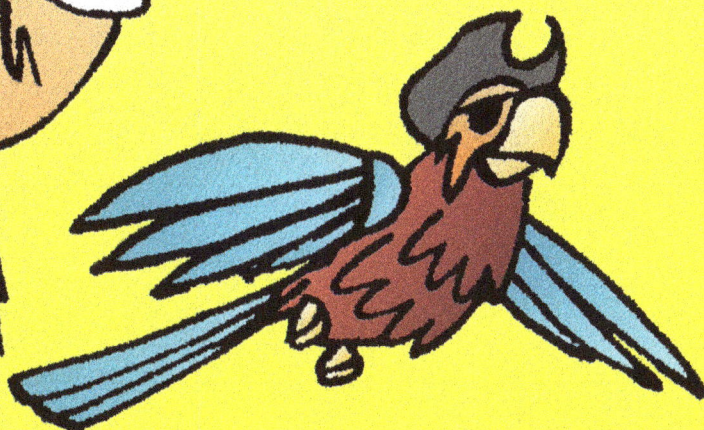

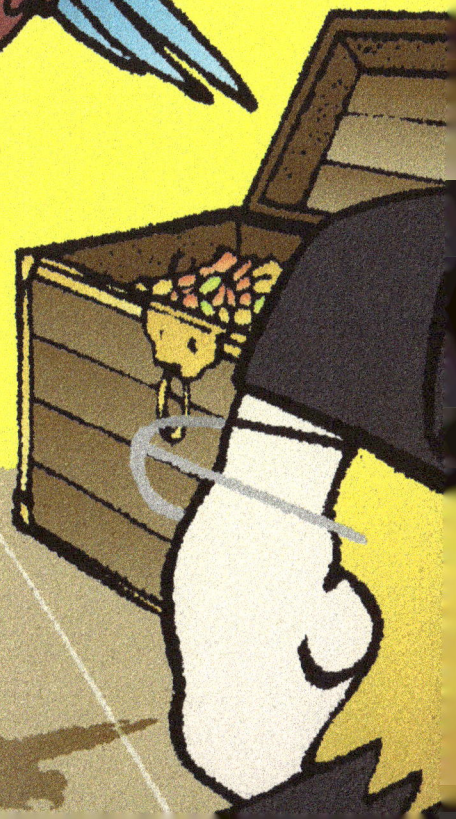

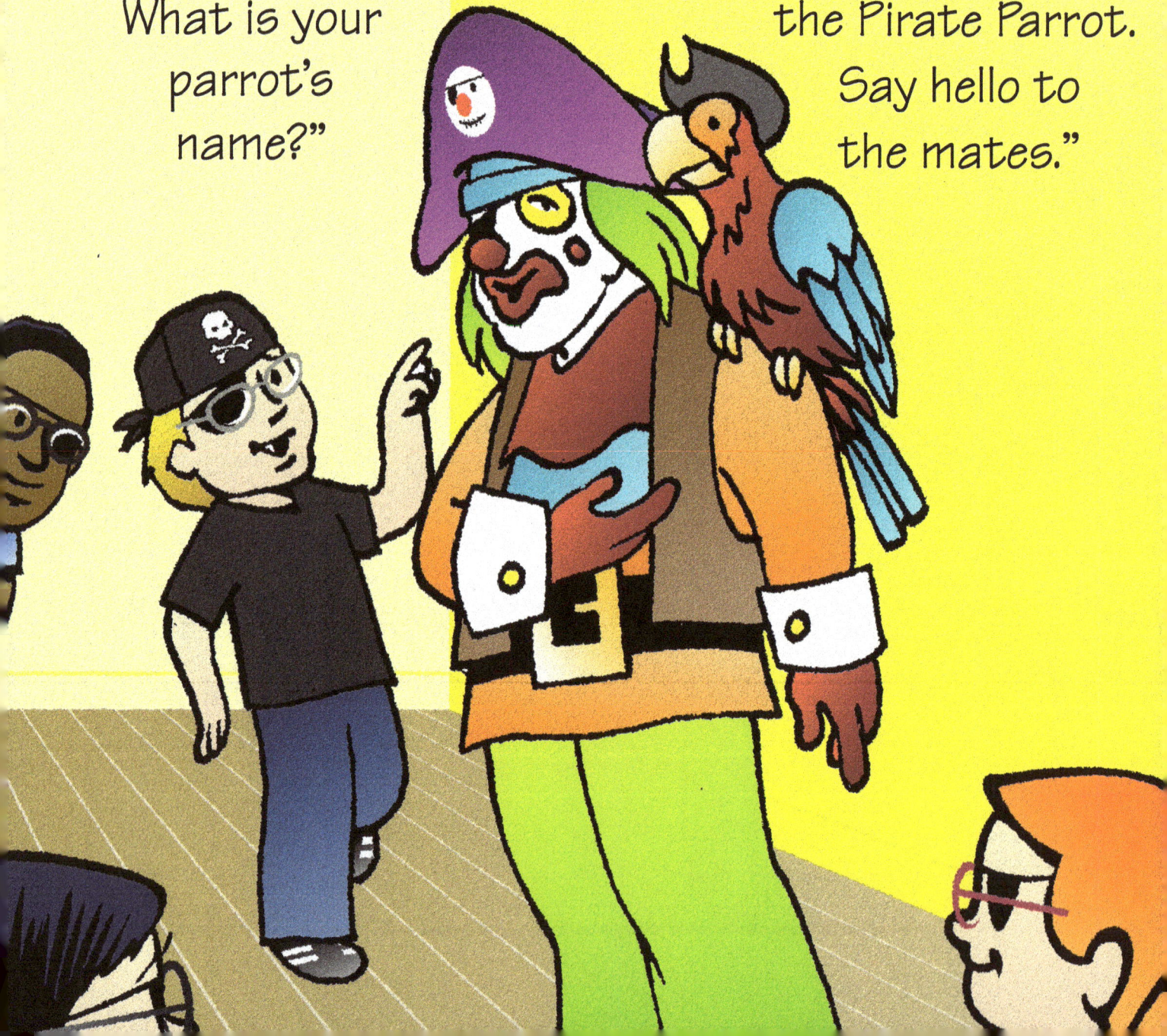

"Hello, Coco the Pirate Clown. What is your parrot's name?"

"Hello, mates. This is Sporty the Pirate Parrot. Say hello to the mates."

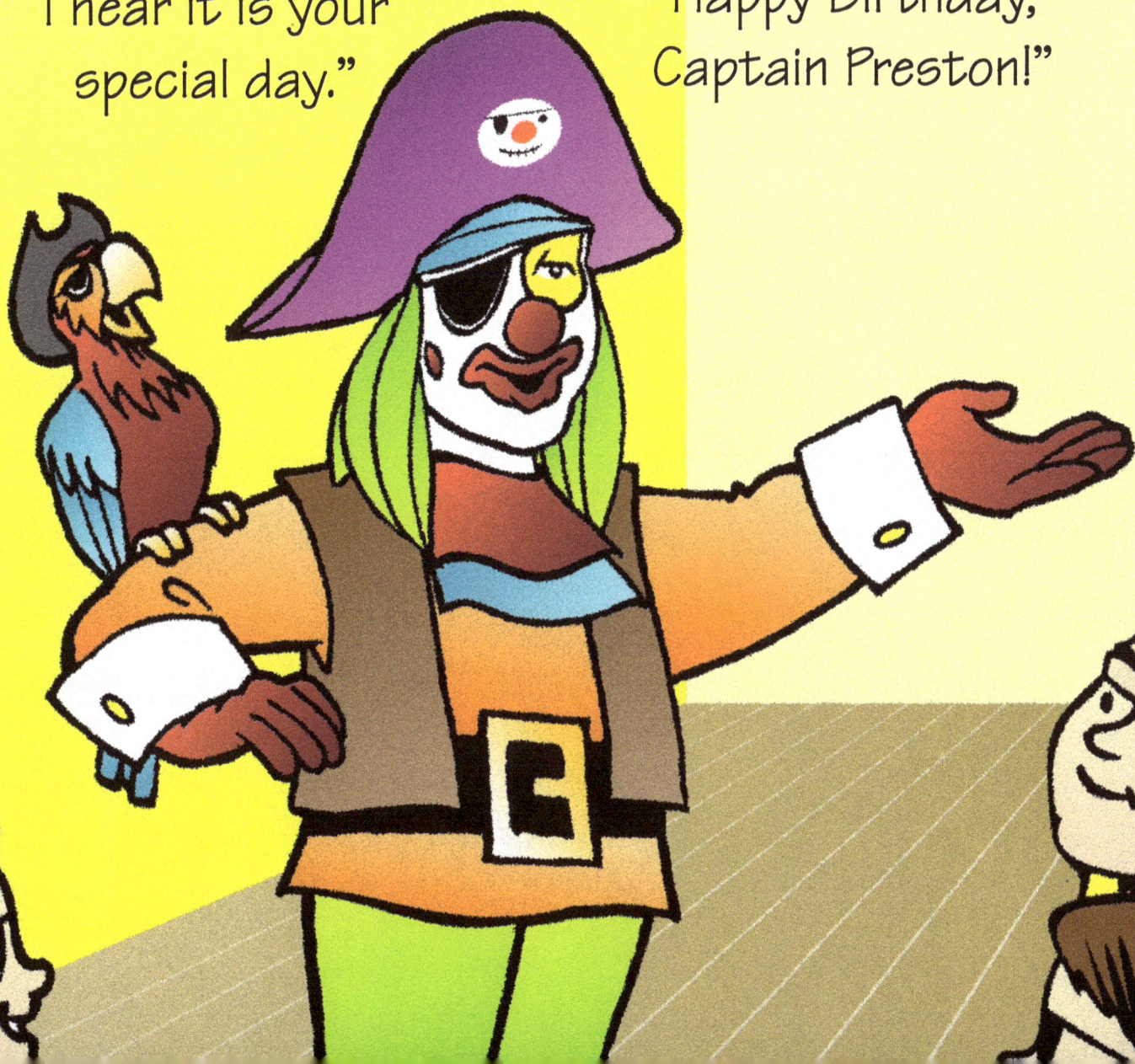

"Hello, mates.
Where is Captain Preston?
I hear it is your
special day."

"Let's all say,
Happy Birthday,
Captain Preston!"

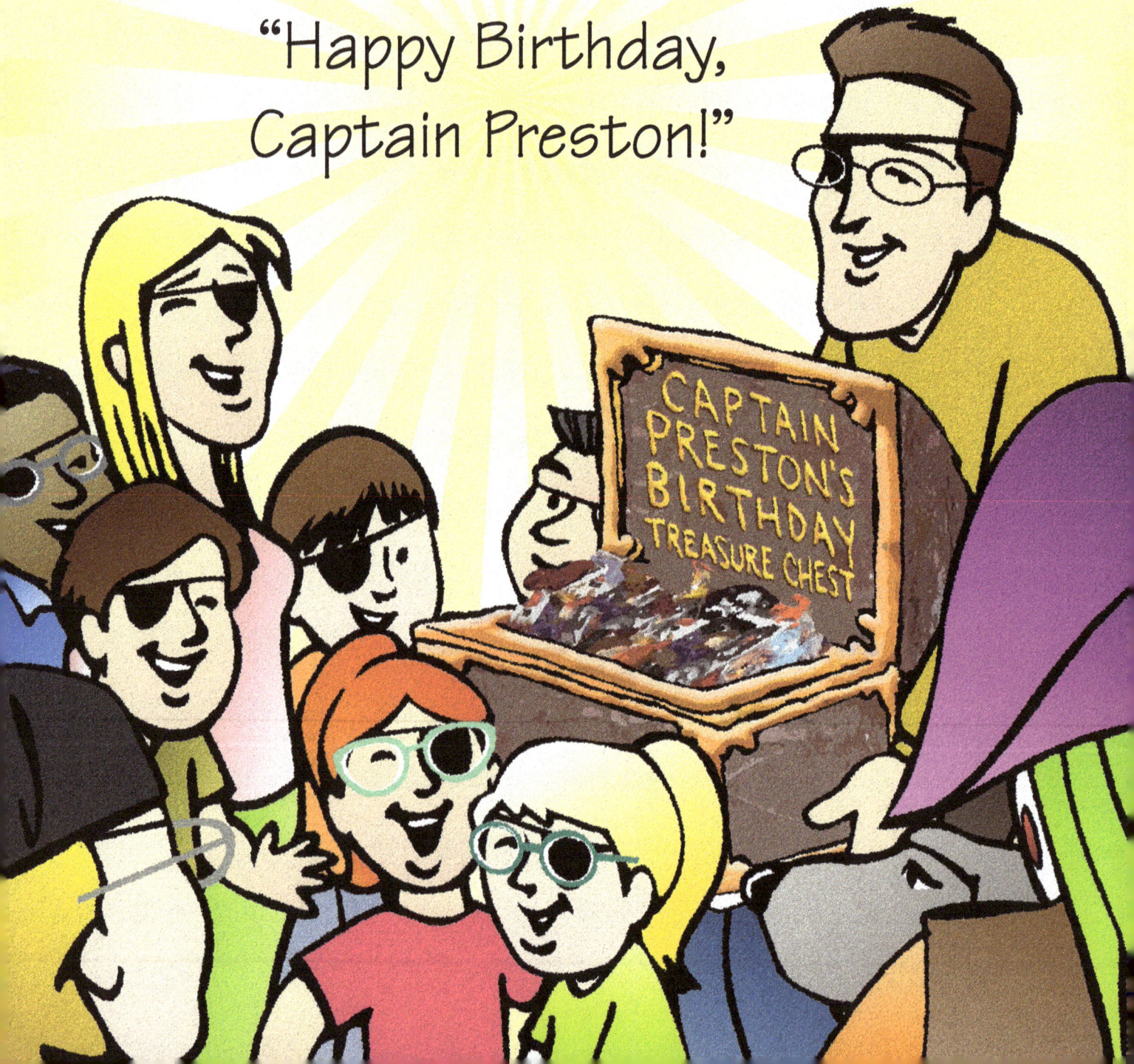

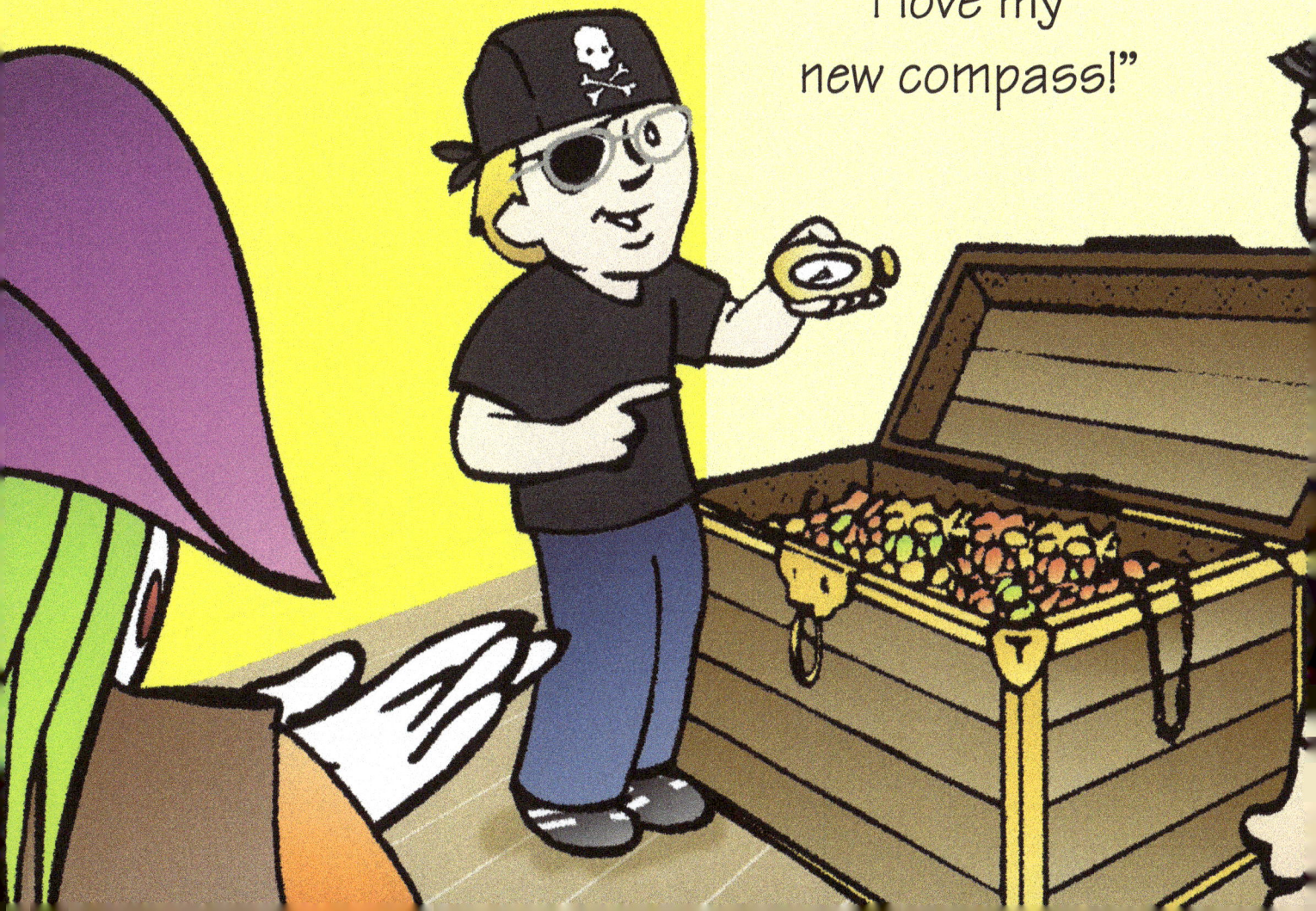

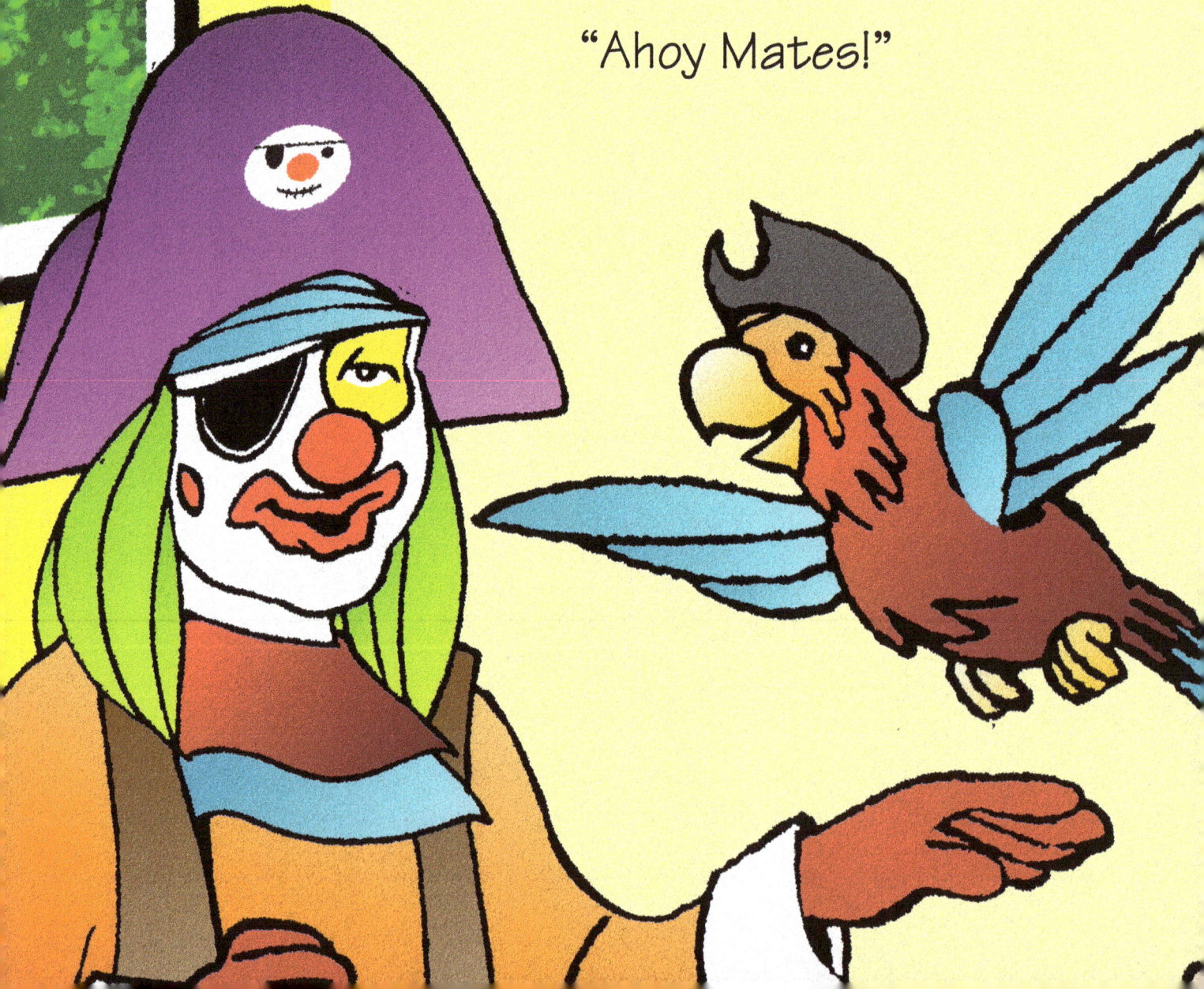

"Mates, it is time for us to go.
Enjoy your treasure and adventure."

"Ahoy Mates!"

"Captain Preston, it is time for you and your shipmates to go outside with the map and compass and find the hidden treasure. I hear there are gold coins."

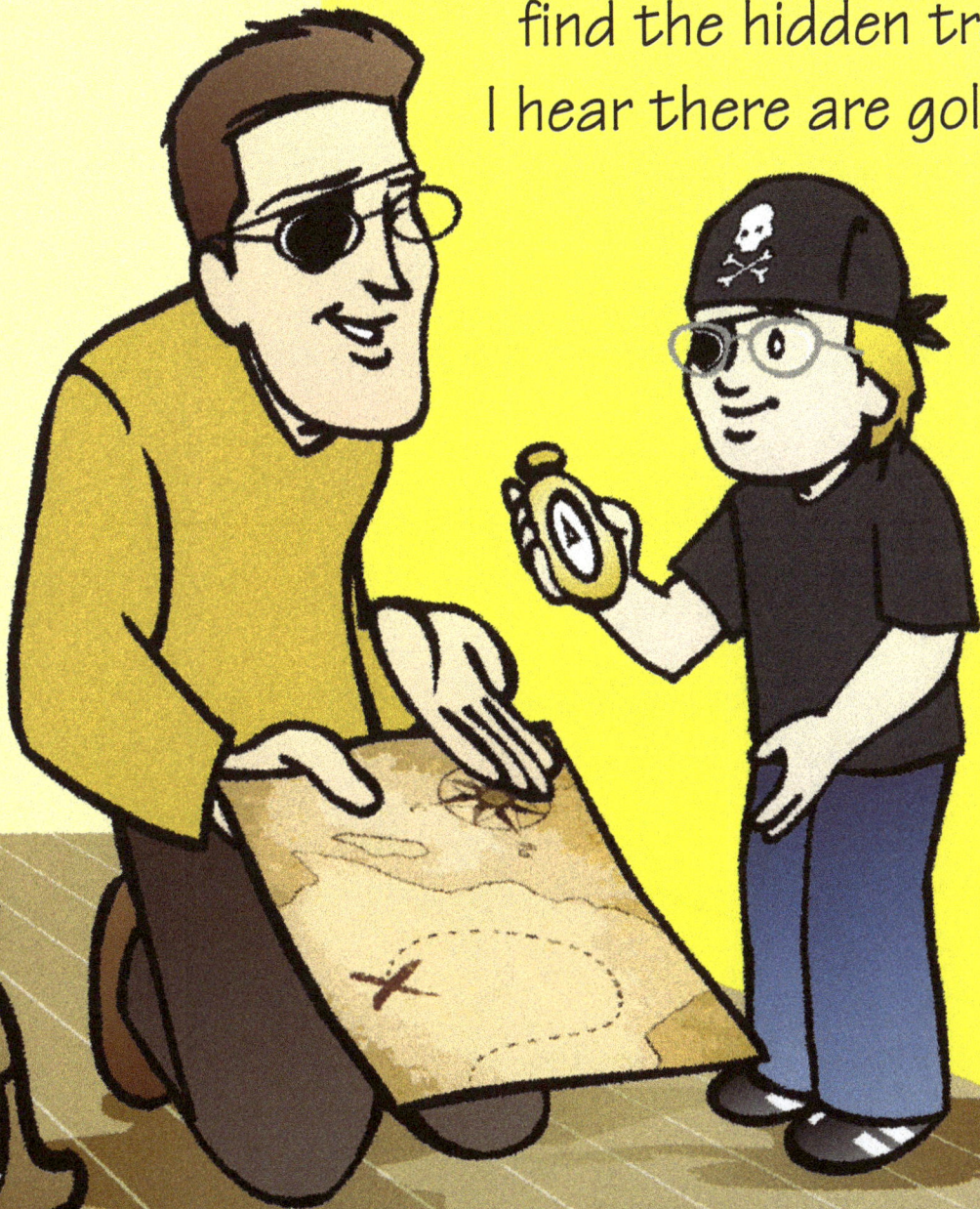

"Okay, Dad, we are
off to our adventure!
We will find the spot
that is marked
on the map
with the big X."

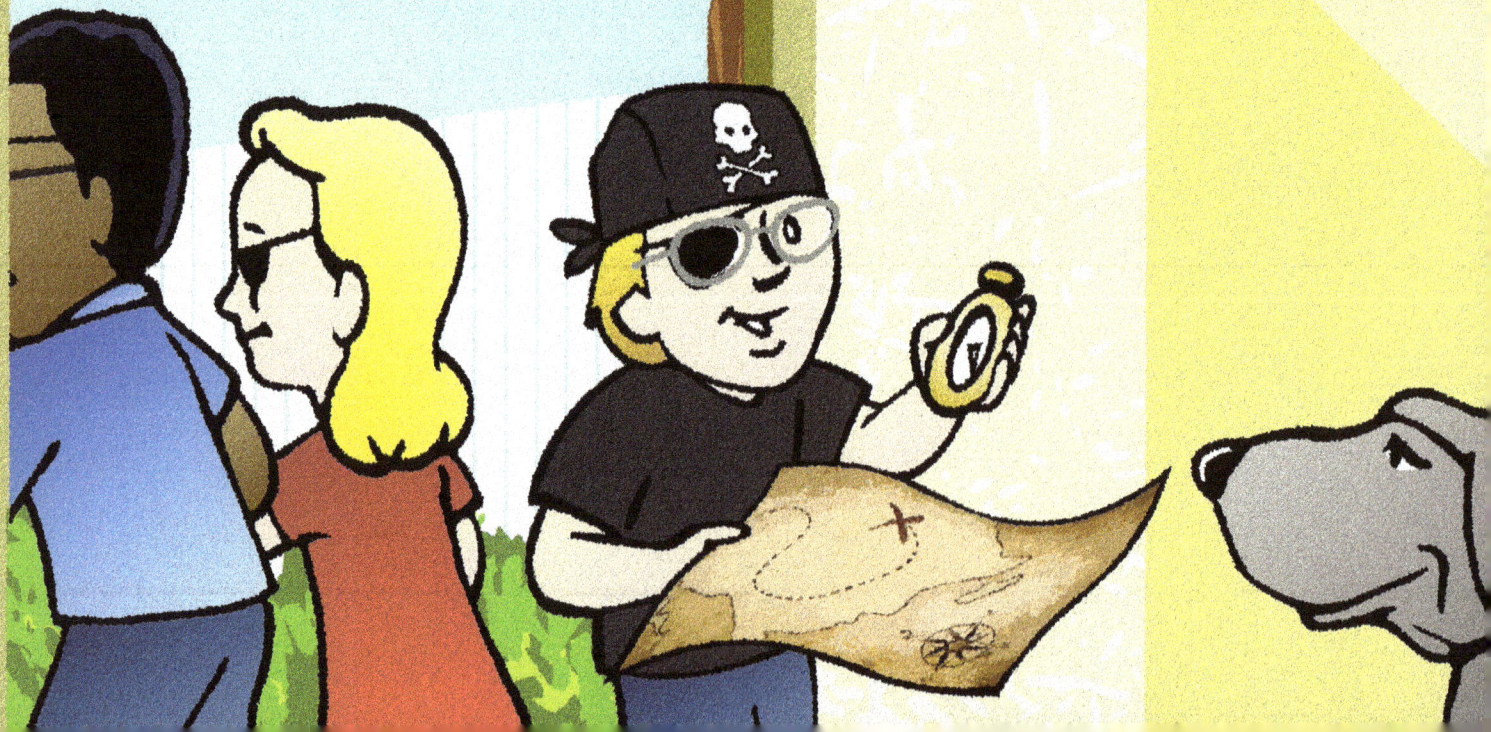

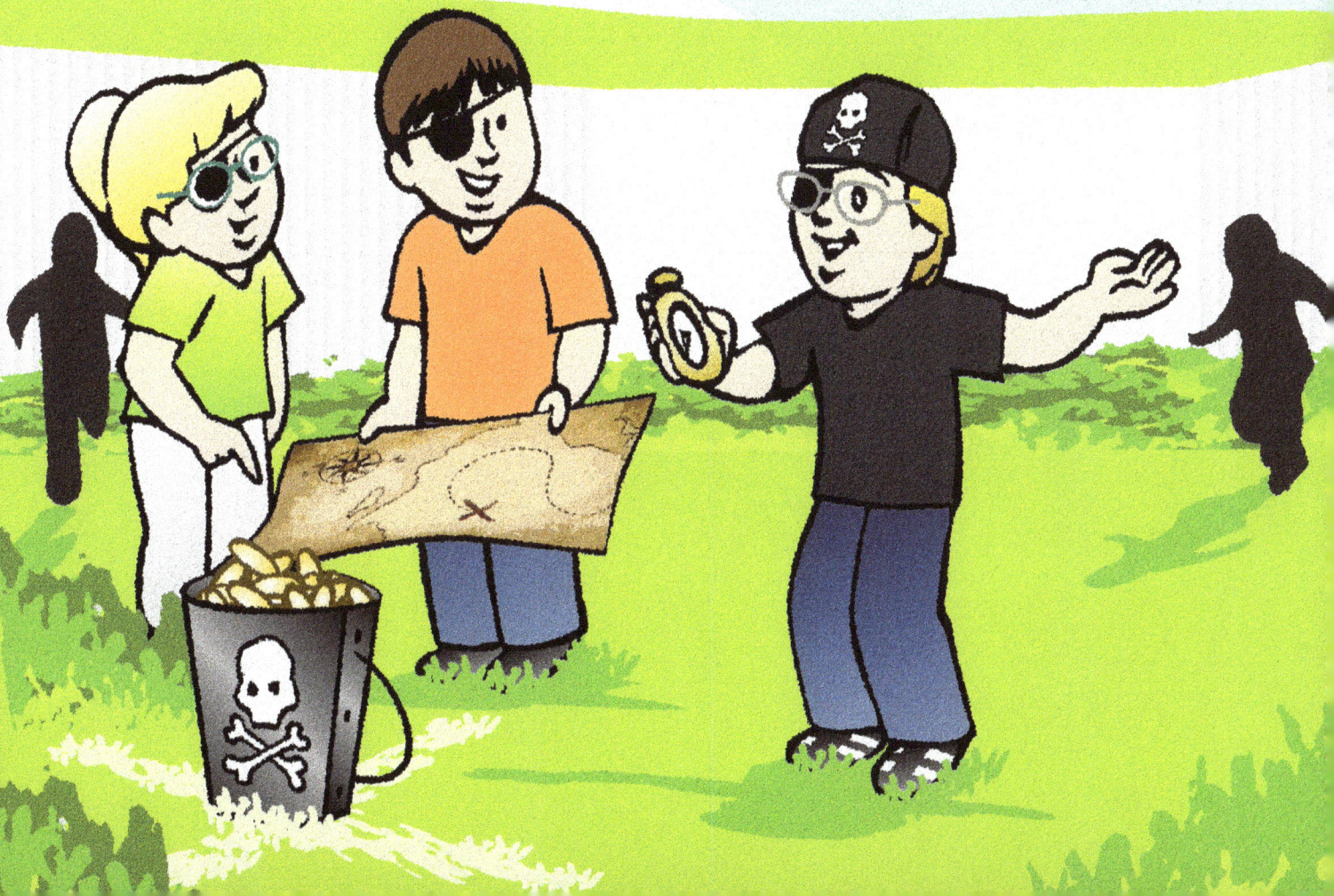

"Look at all of our treasures!"

"See, Captain Preston, you and your shipmates can do anything with your eye patches on."

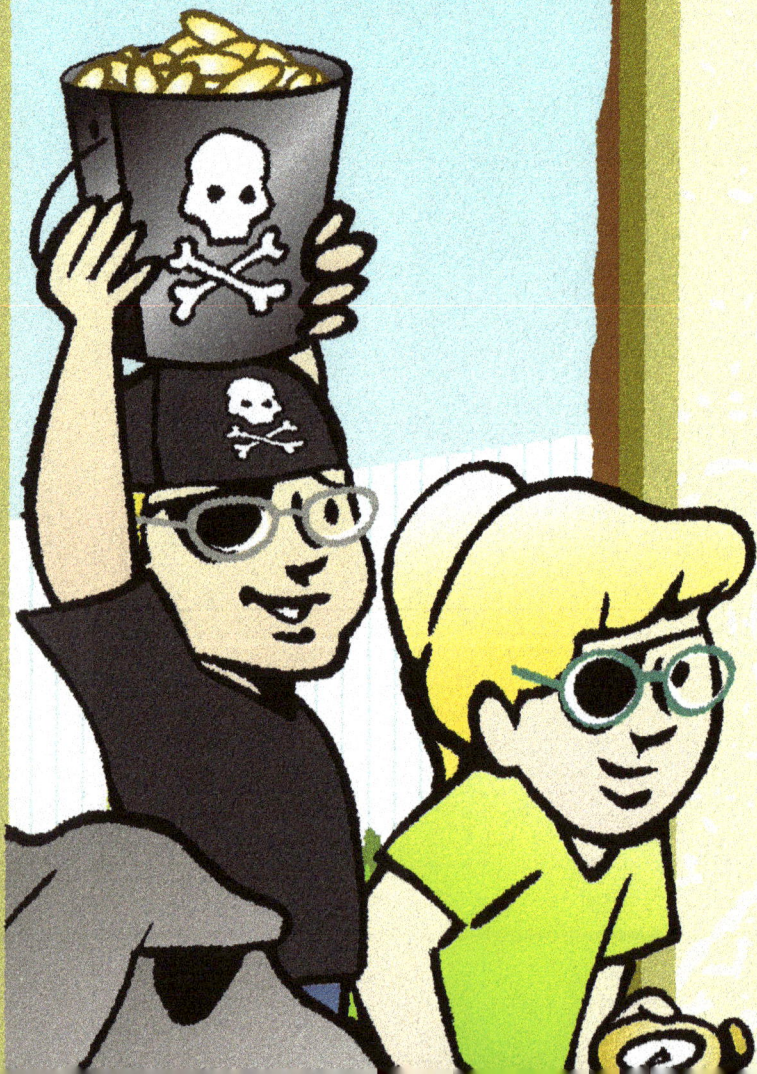

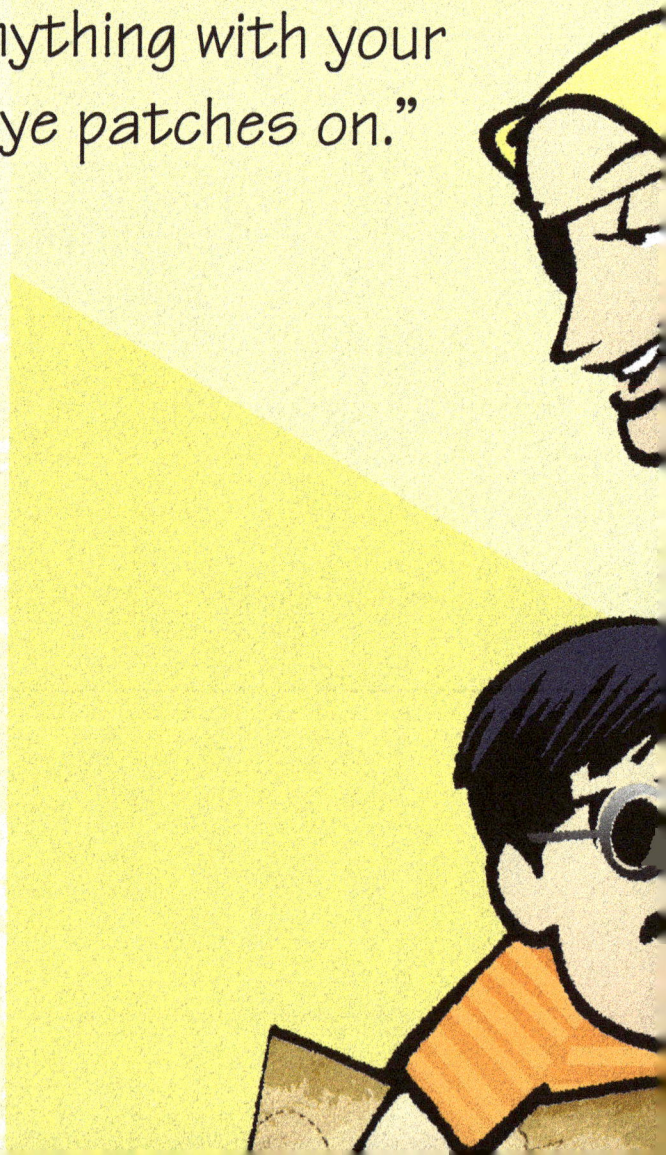

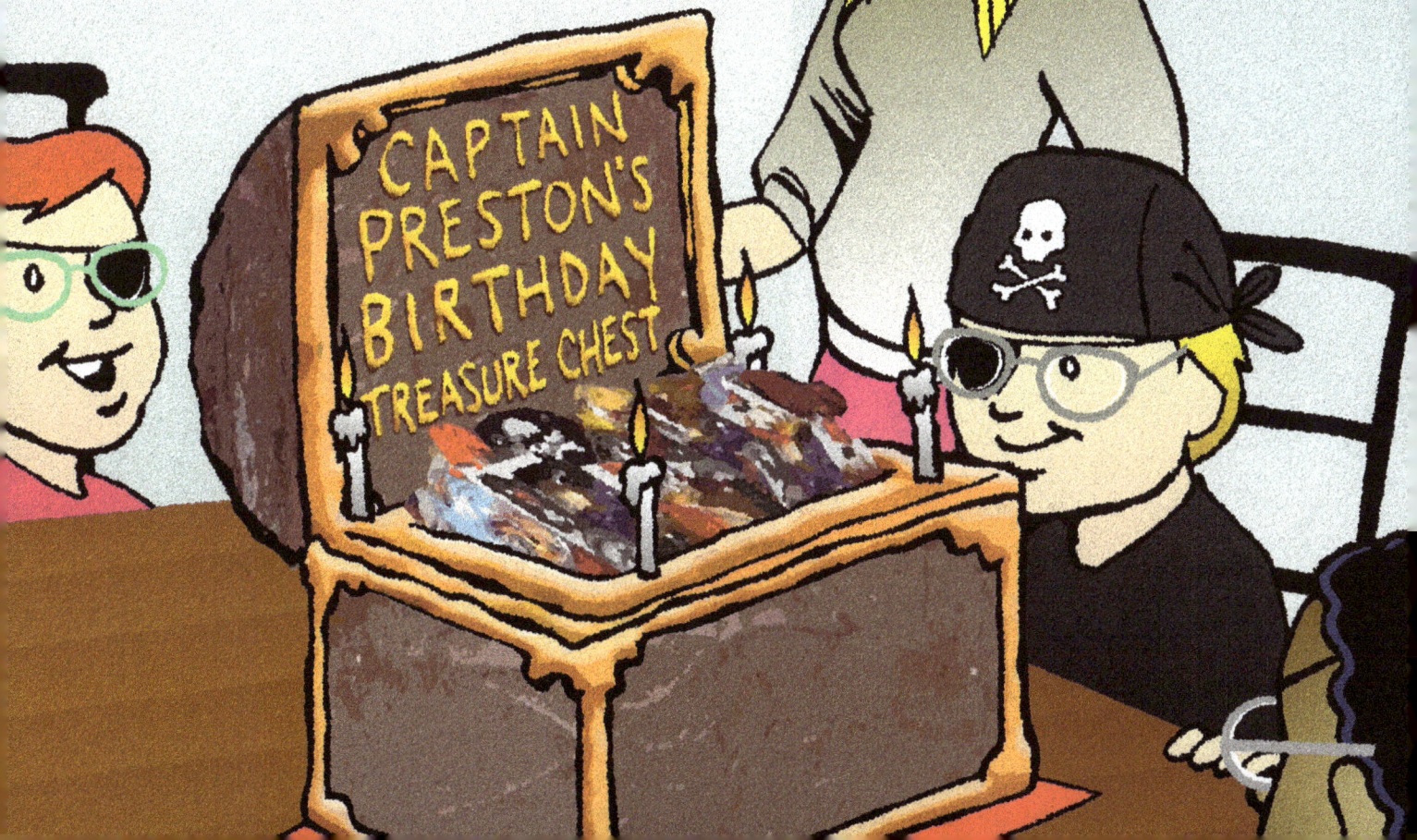

"Mates, we need to sing now!
Happy birthday
dear Captain Preston!
Happy birthday to you!"

"Now make a wish and
blow out the candles!"

CAPTAIN PRESTON'S BIRTHDAY TREASURE CHEST

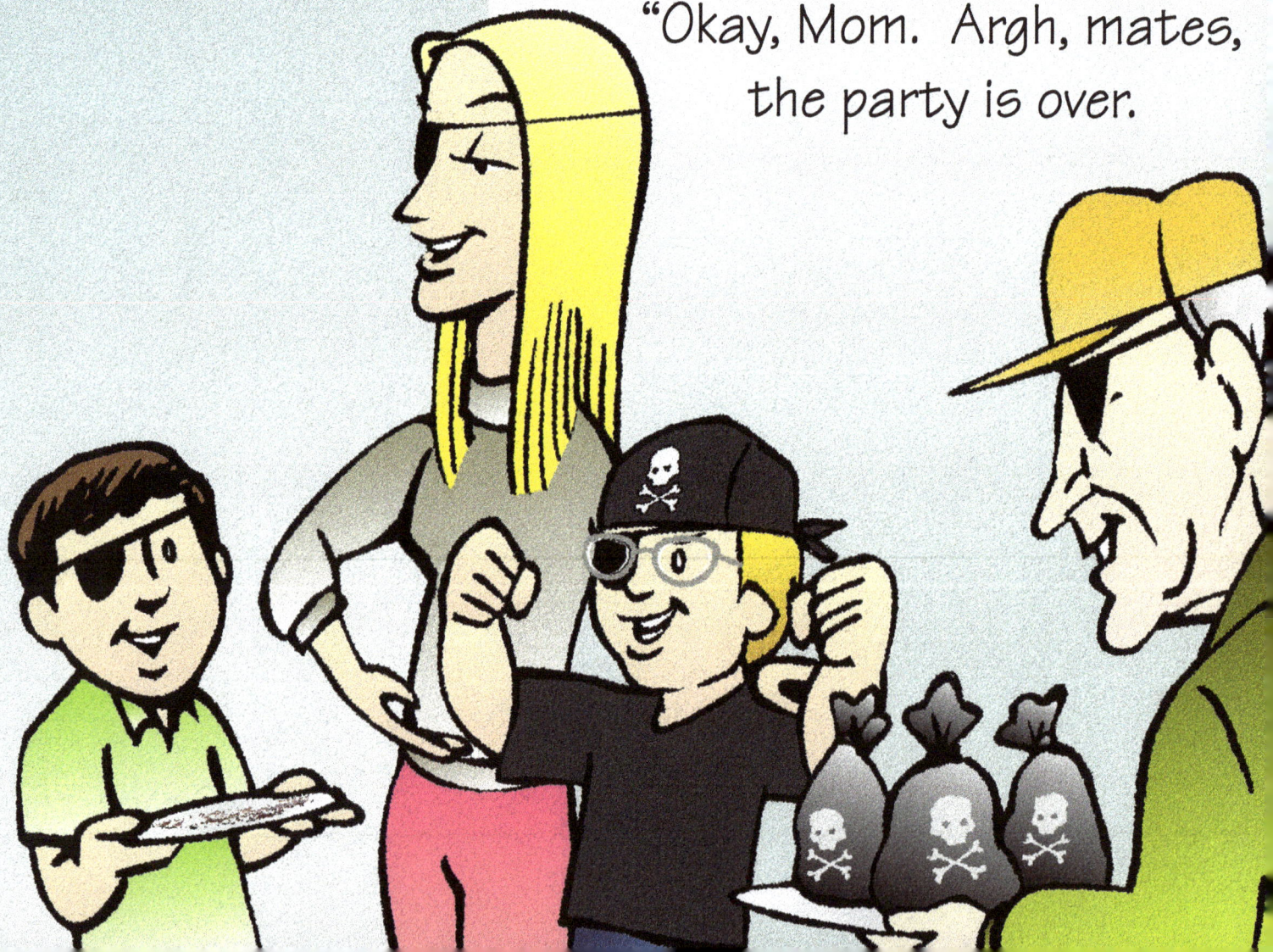

"Captain Preston, it has been a long day. I am very proud of you for wearing your patch for so long. Now, let's get ready for bed so you can go to Patch Land."

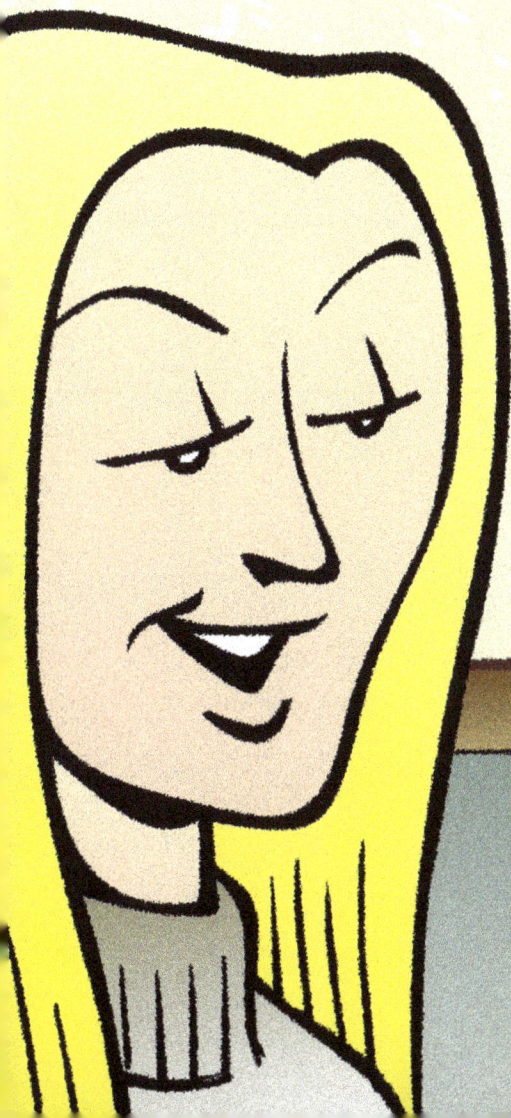

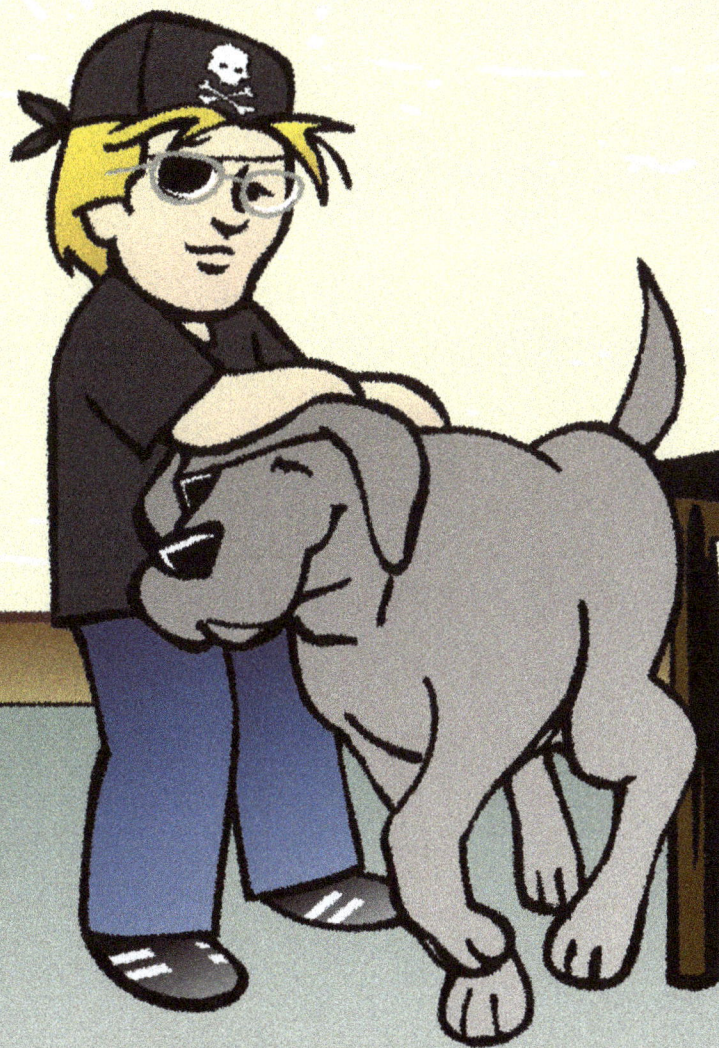

"Let's go to sleep Beau. I am excited to see who will show up in Patch Land tonight."

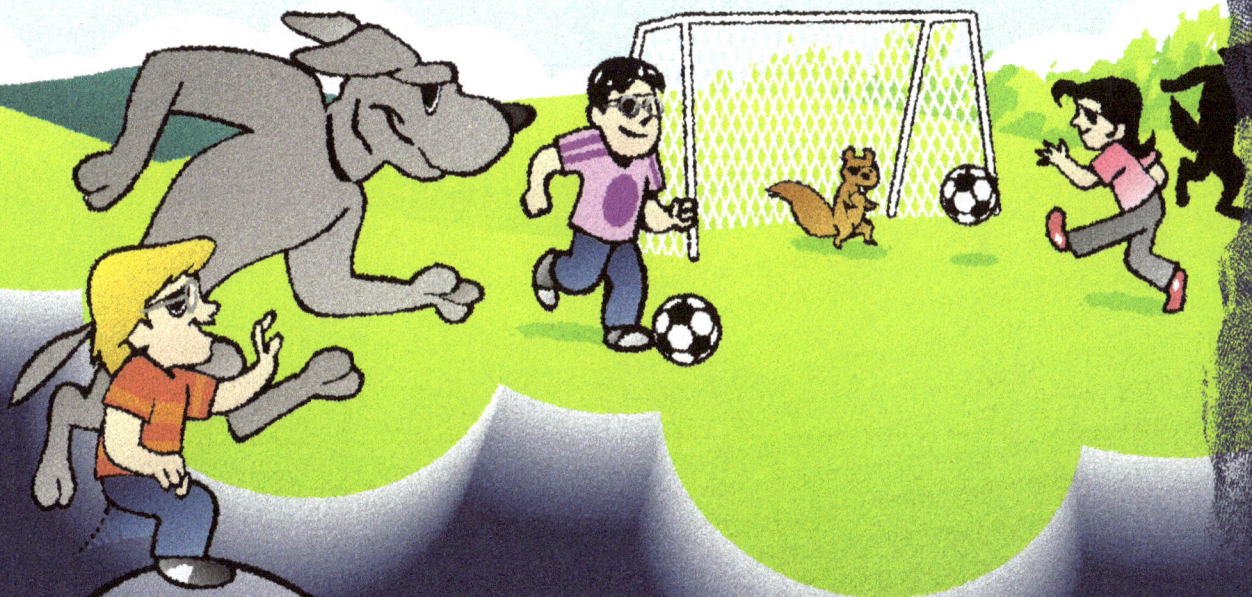
"Here we are, Beau, in Patch Land. Our friends are waiting for us to play soccer. Hello, Tommy. You decided to come again."

"Yes I did! I wanted to tell you that my doctor told me that my eye is doing better! She said for me to keep up the good work!"

"I told you it worked!"

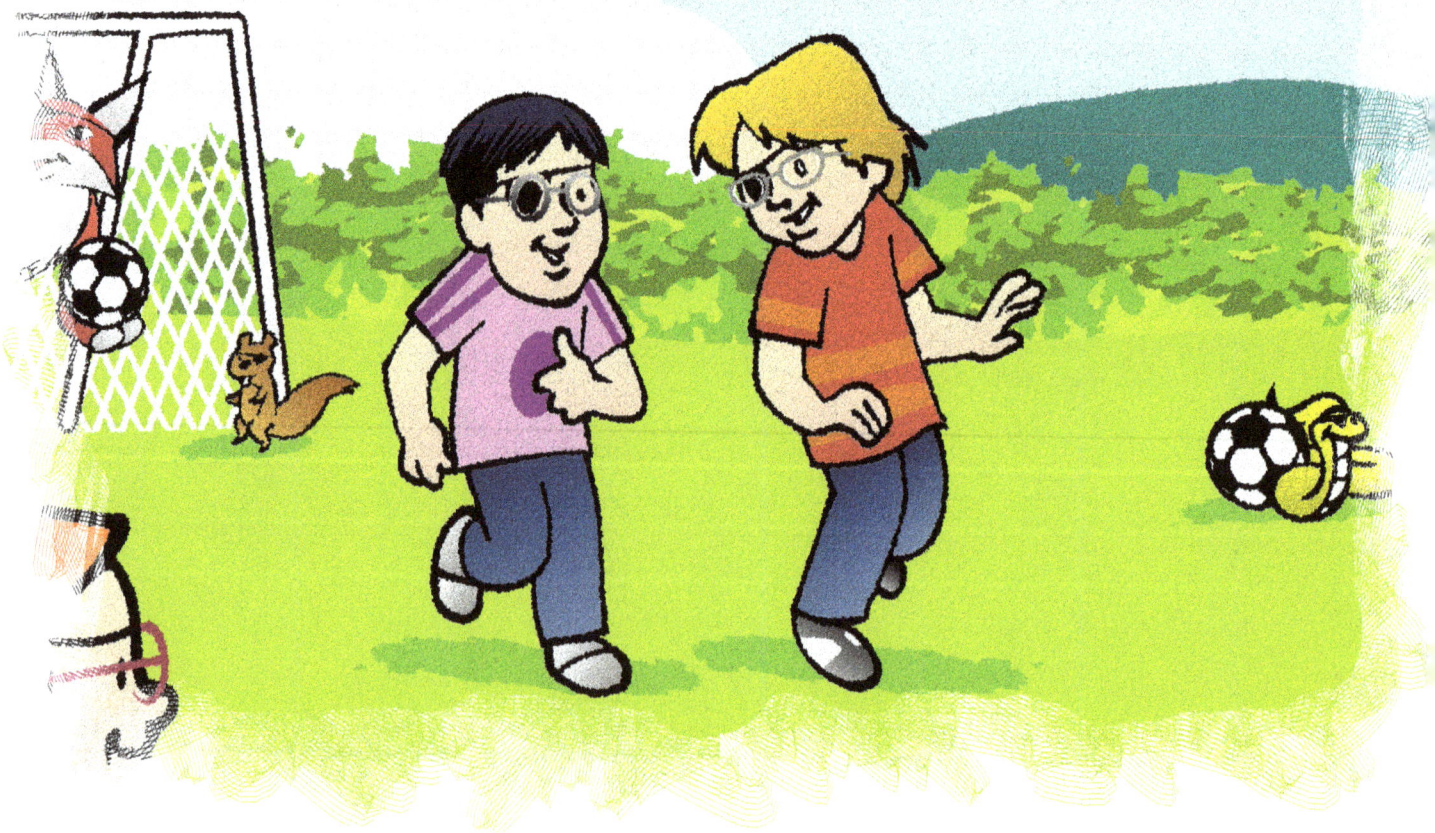

"Did you want to play soccer with us? You can be on the other team. We already have our team. We have Missy our neighbor, Banjo the bengal tiger, Snort the pig, Pepe the malamute, Foxy the fox, Peetree the squirrel, and my favorite horse, Winston. Oh, and Baca the German shepherd. He is really good. We also picked Thor the Great Dane."

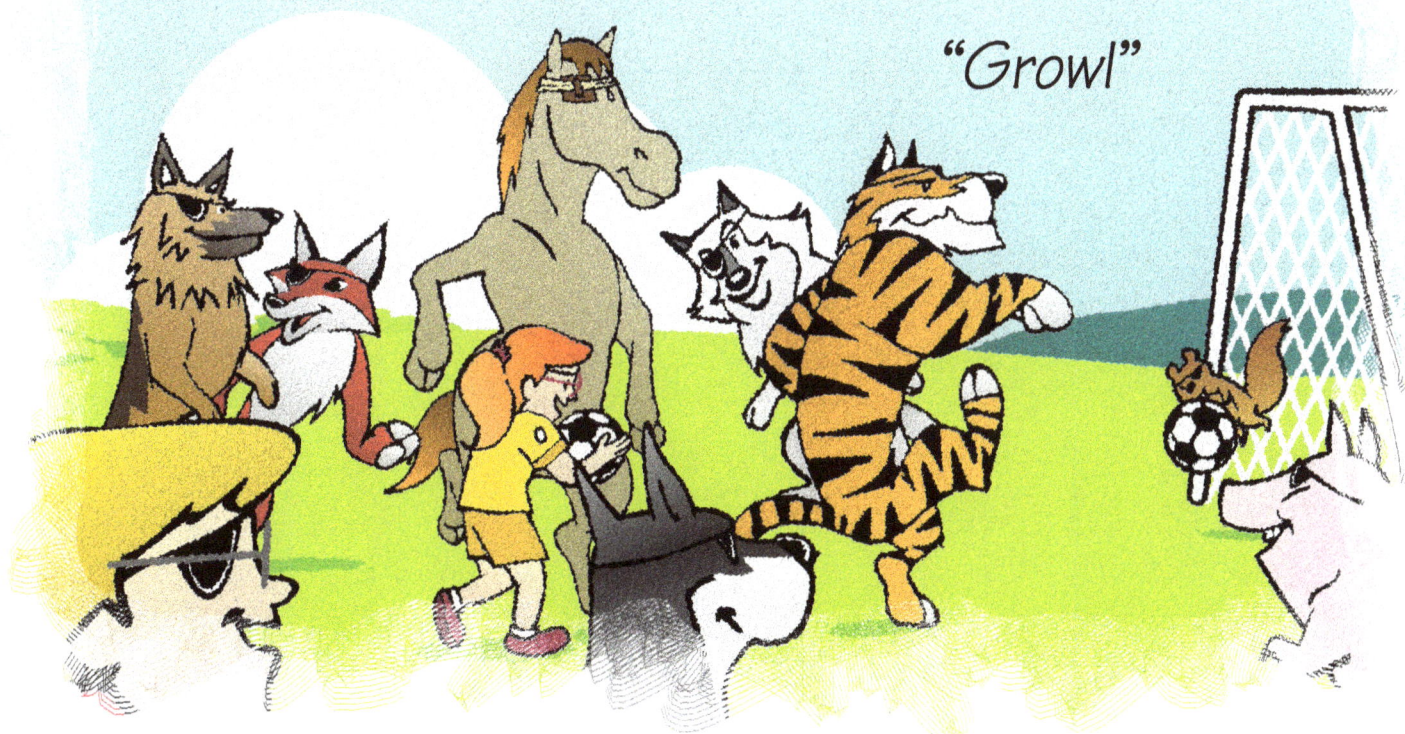

"Growl"

"Tommy, you also have really good players on your team. Let's go meet them. Here is Billy, Bentley the old English sheep dog, Stinky the skunk, and your best player, Beau. Stryker the golden dog and Beery the black bear, Slinky the snake, Manny the mini dashund, and let's not forget Won Ton the small black and white dog. Won Ton, he is fast!"

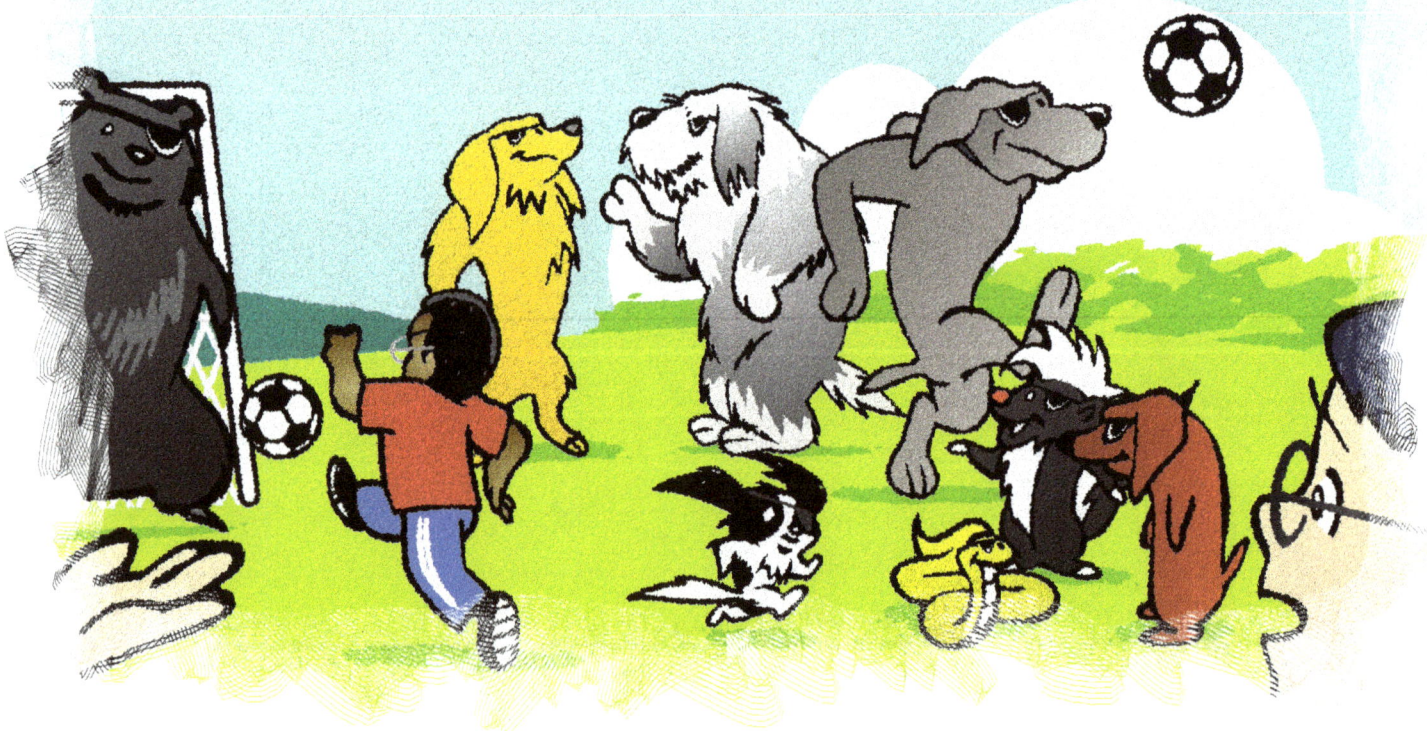

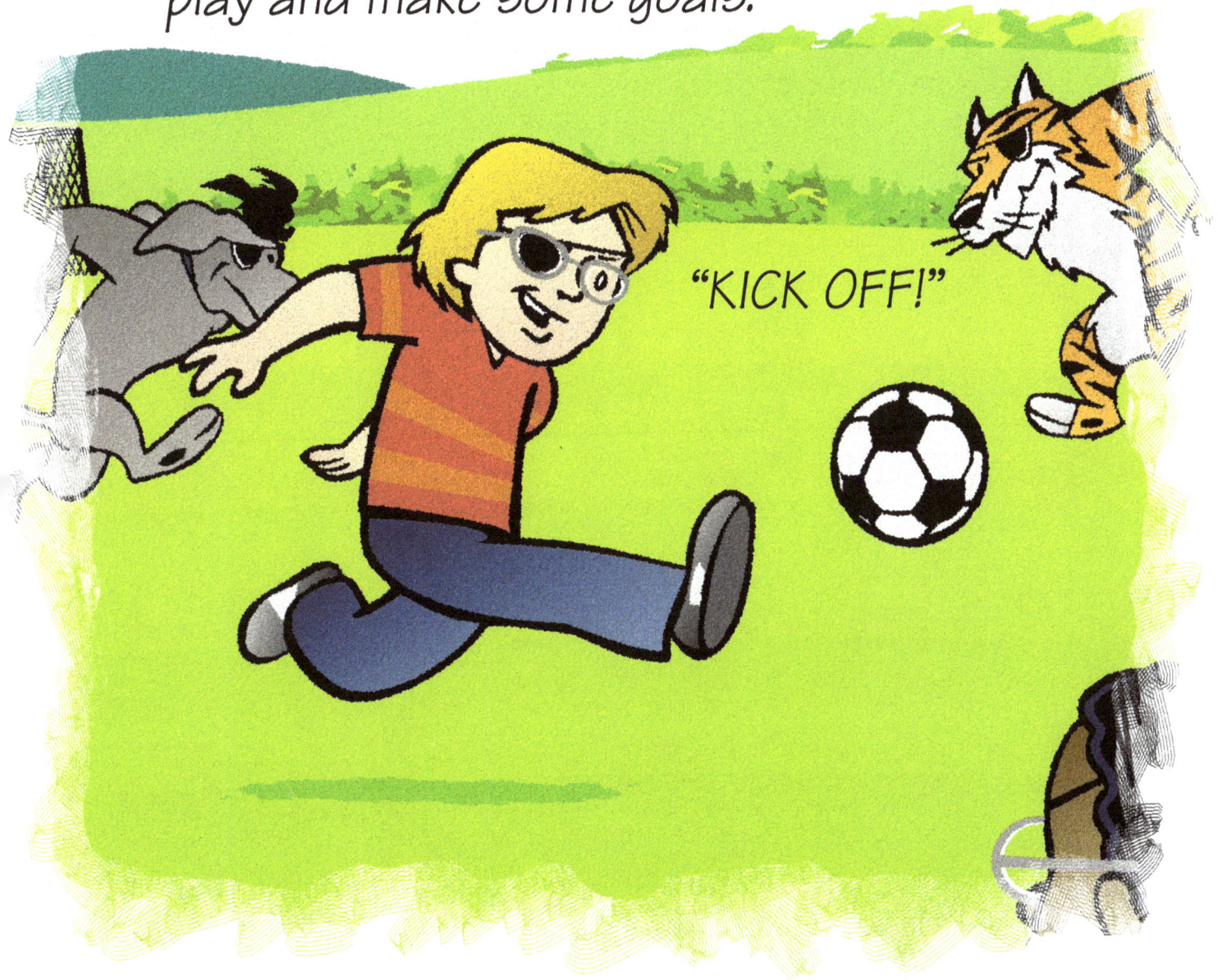

"Beau got the ball.
Run, Beau, Run!
Oh, no. Banjo
just stole the ball."

"He passed it
to Missy.
Beery the Black Bear
is trying to
block the goal."

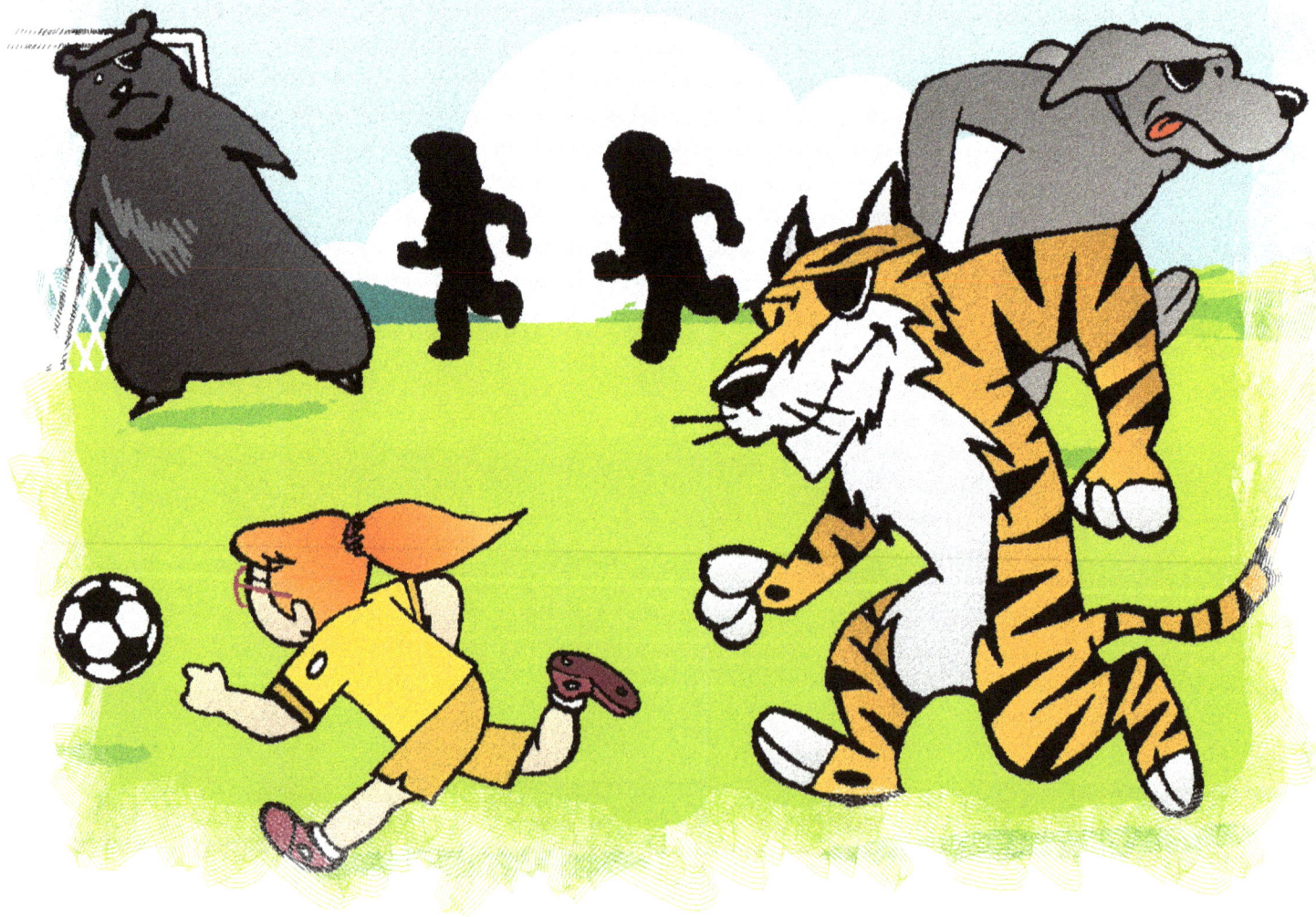

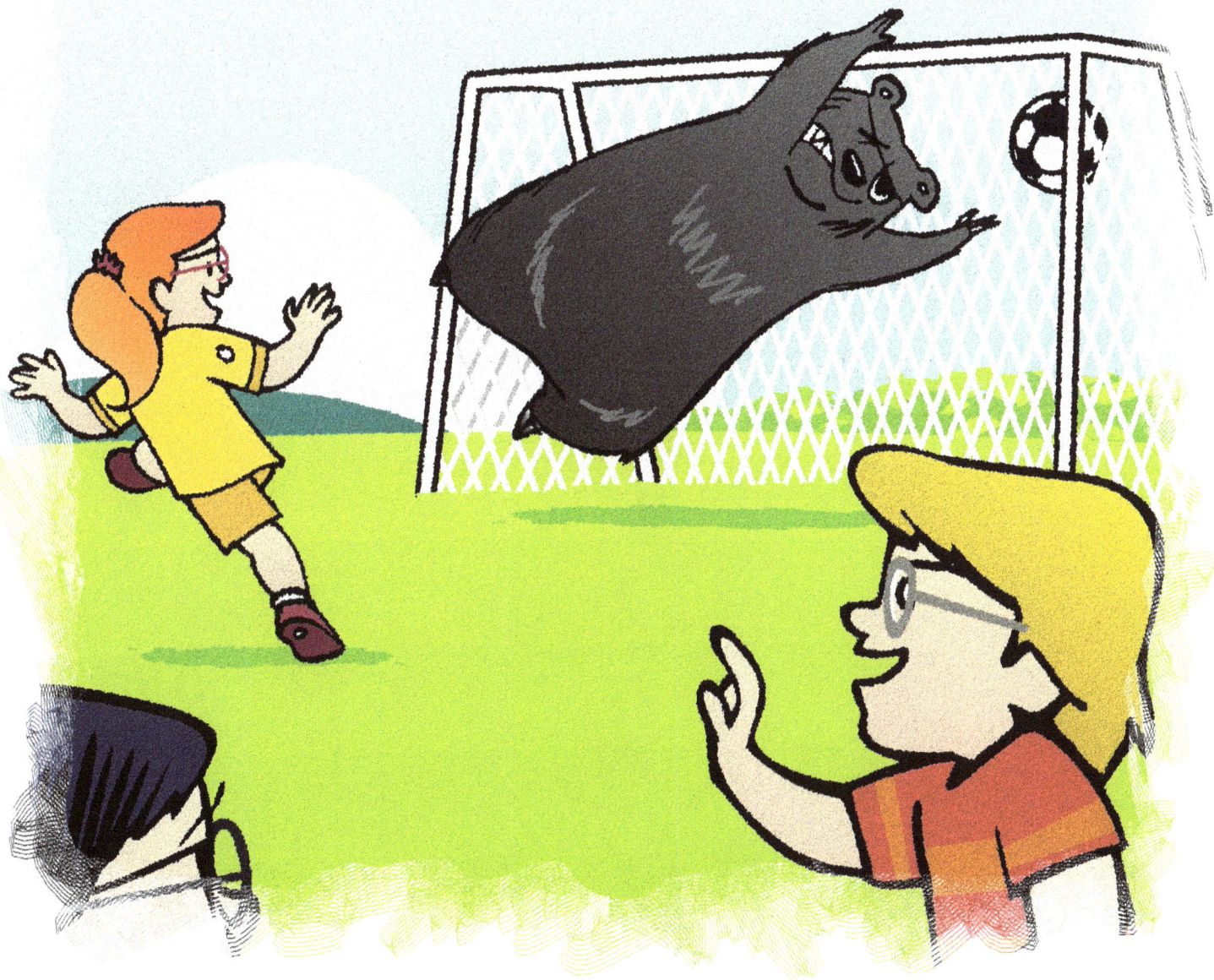

"Good job, Missy. You scored! GOAL! You can do anything with an eye patch on."

"Tommy, I have to go now.
My mom is trying to wake me up.
Bye. I will see you all
later at school."

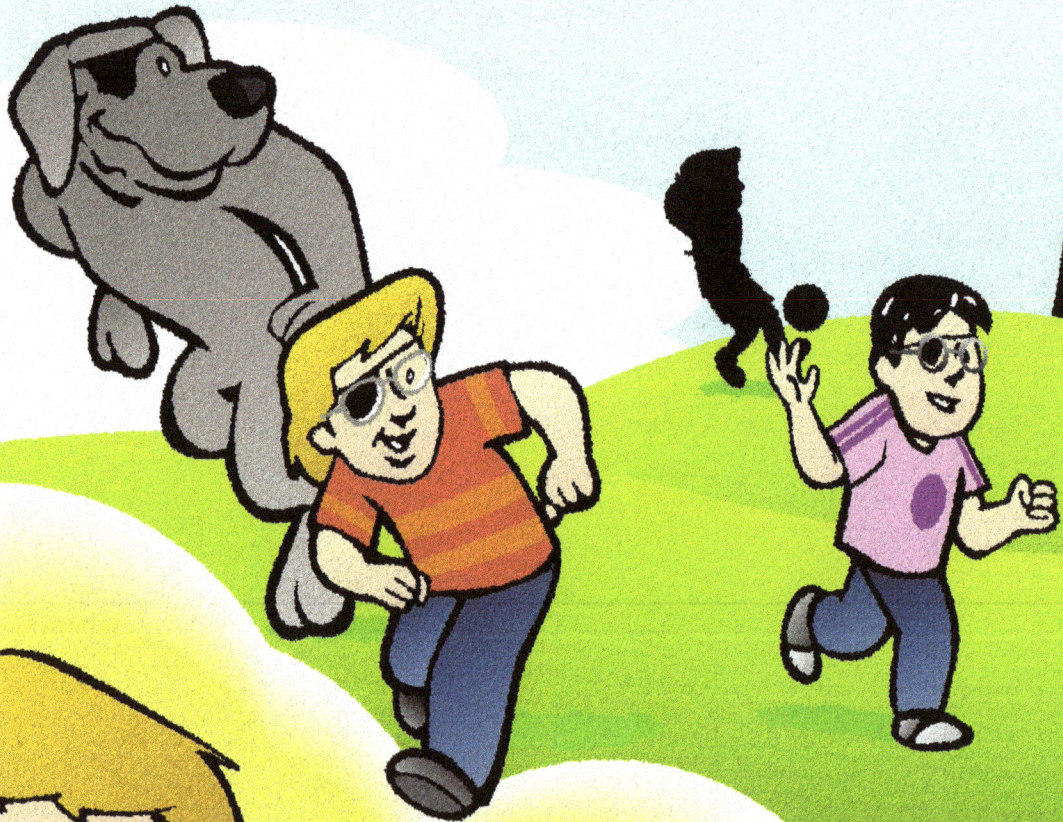

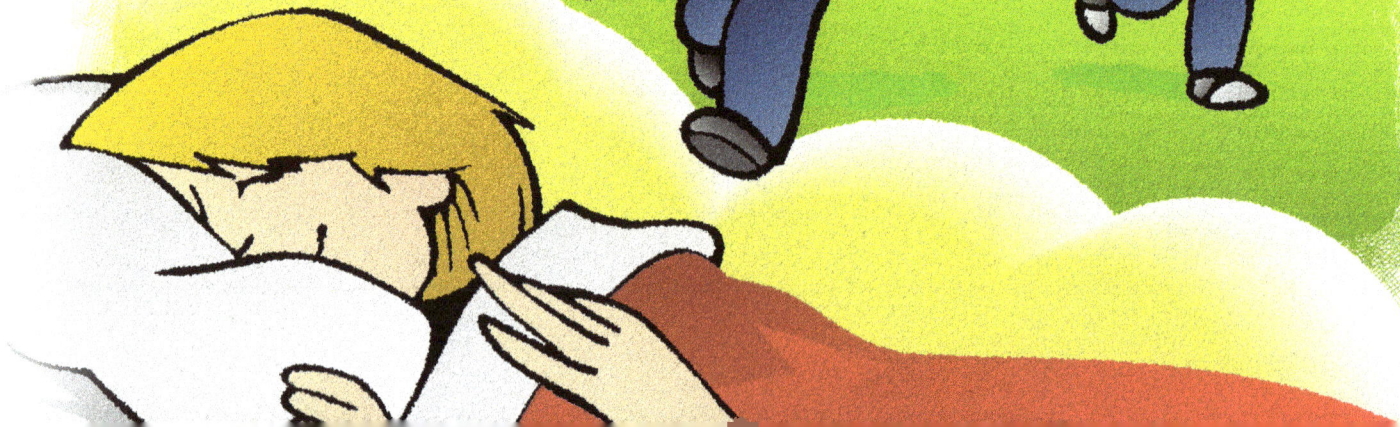

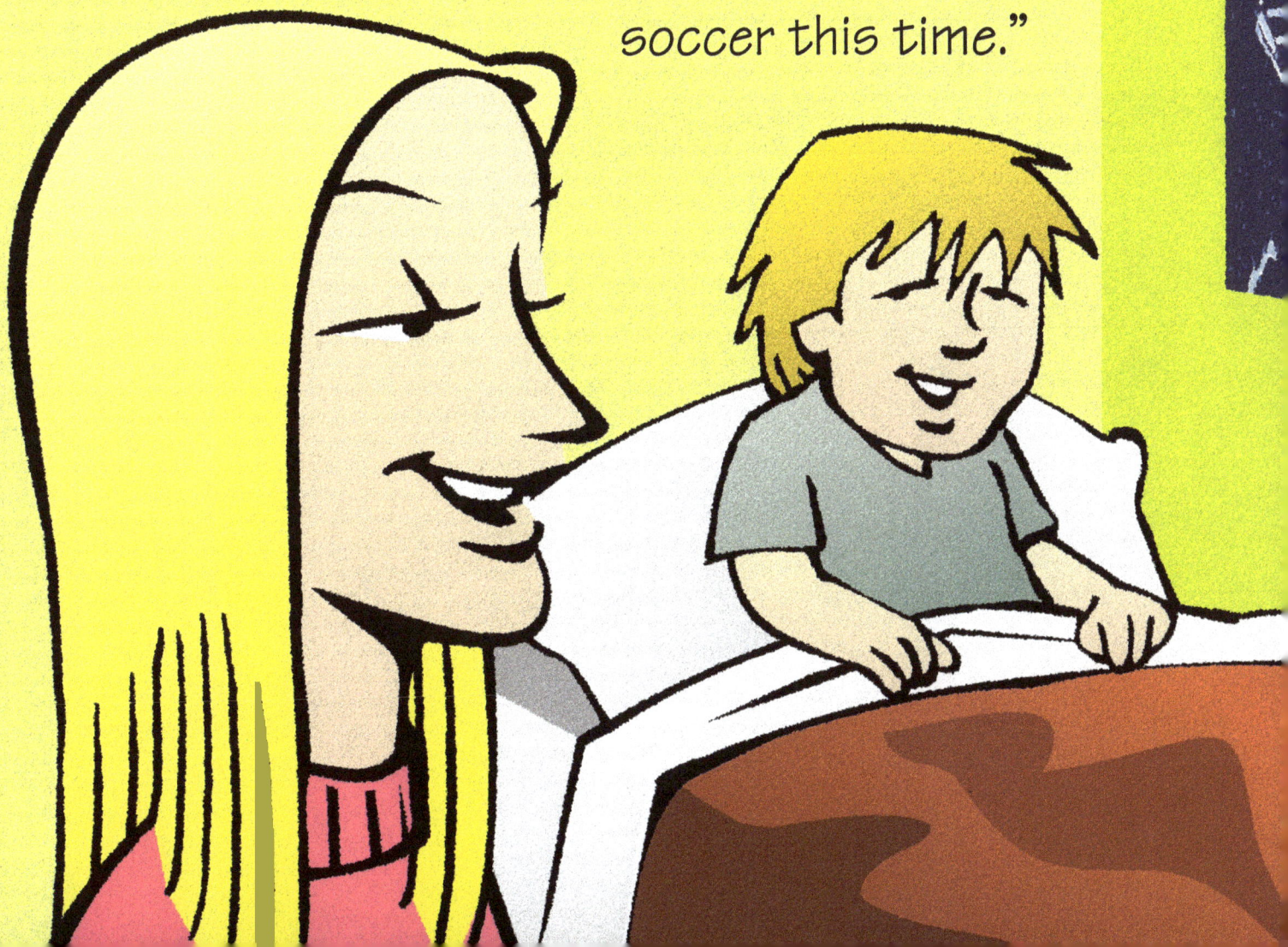

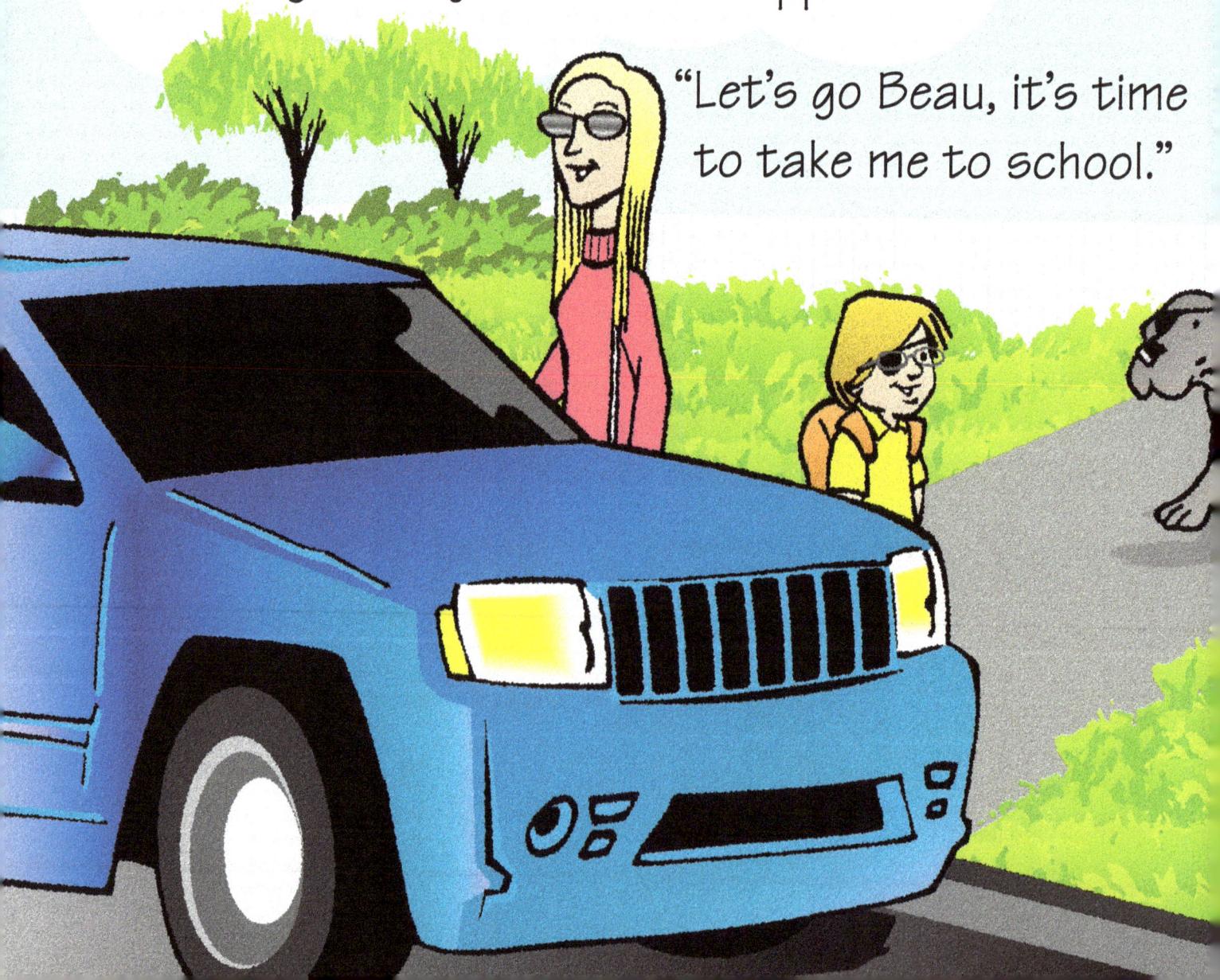

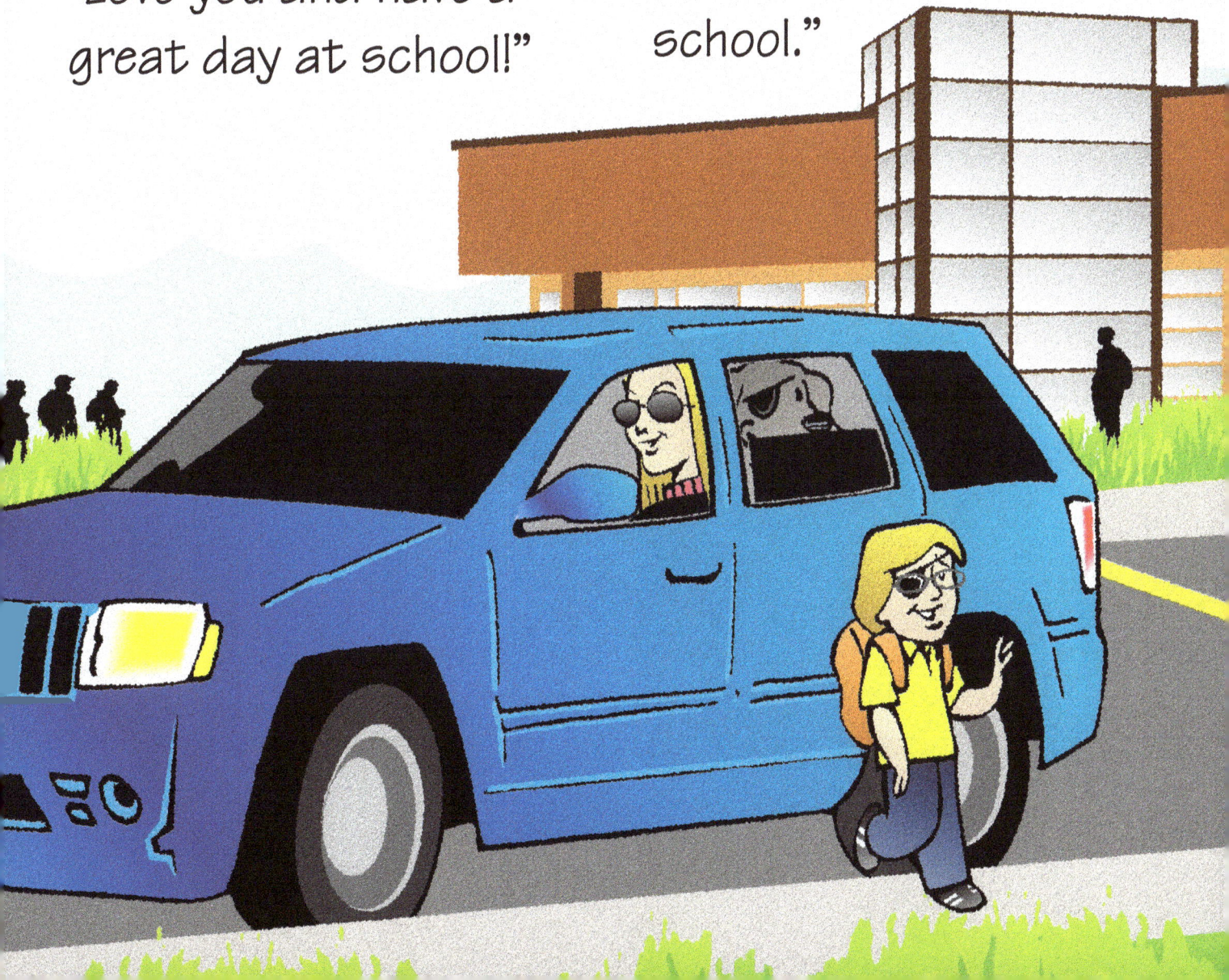

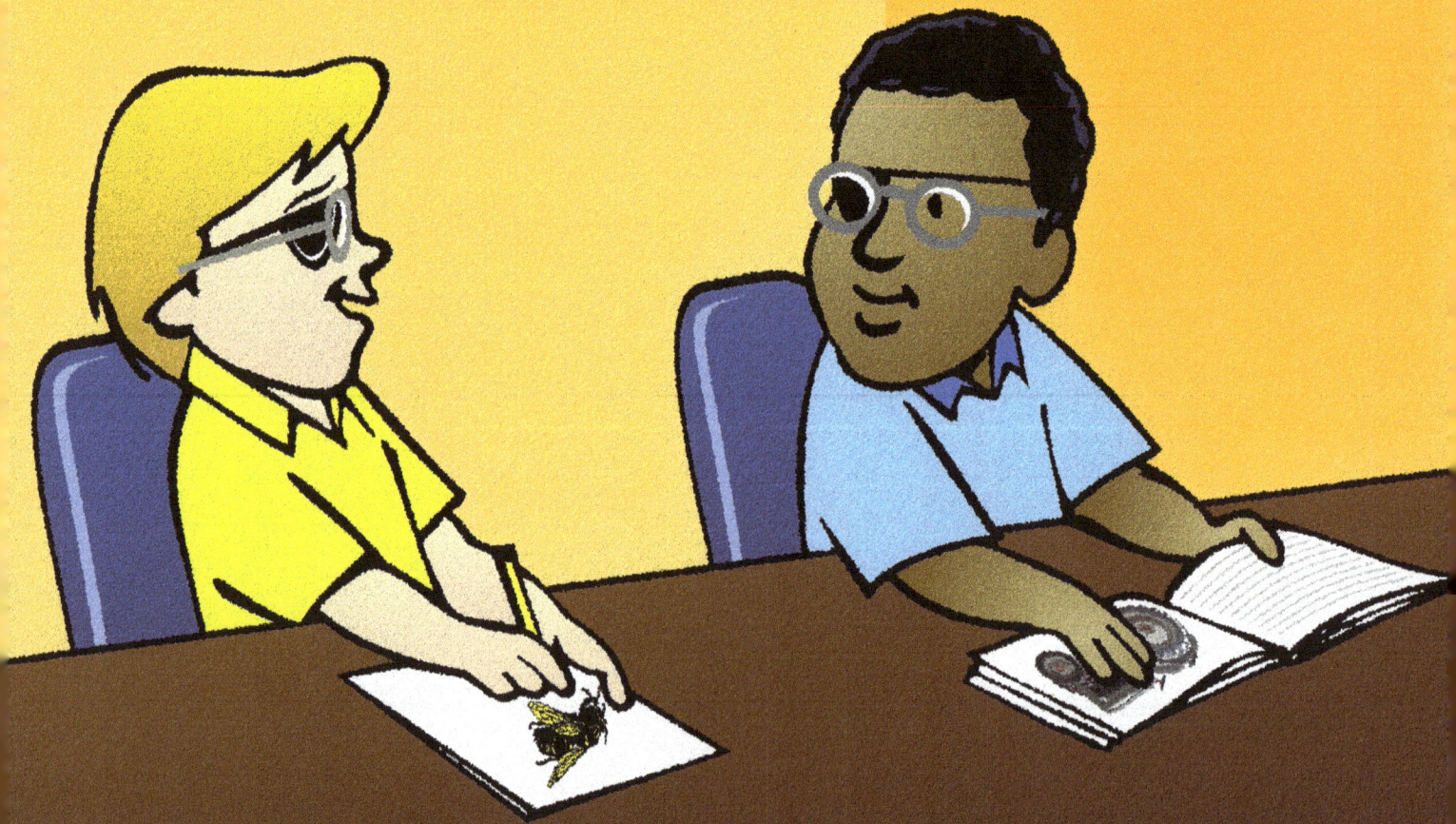

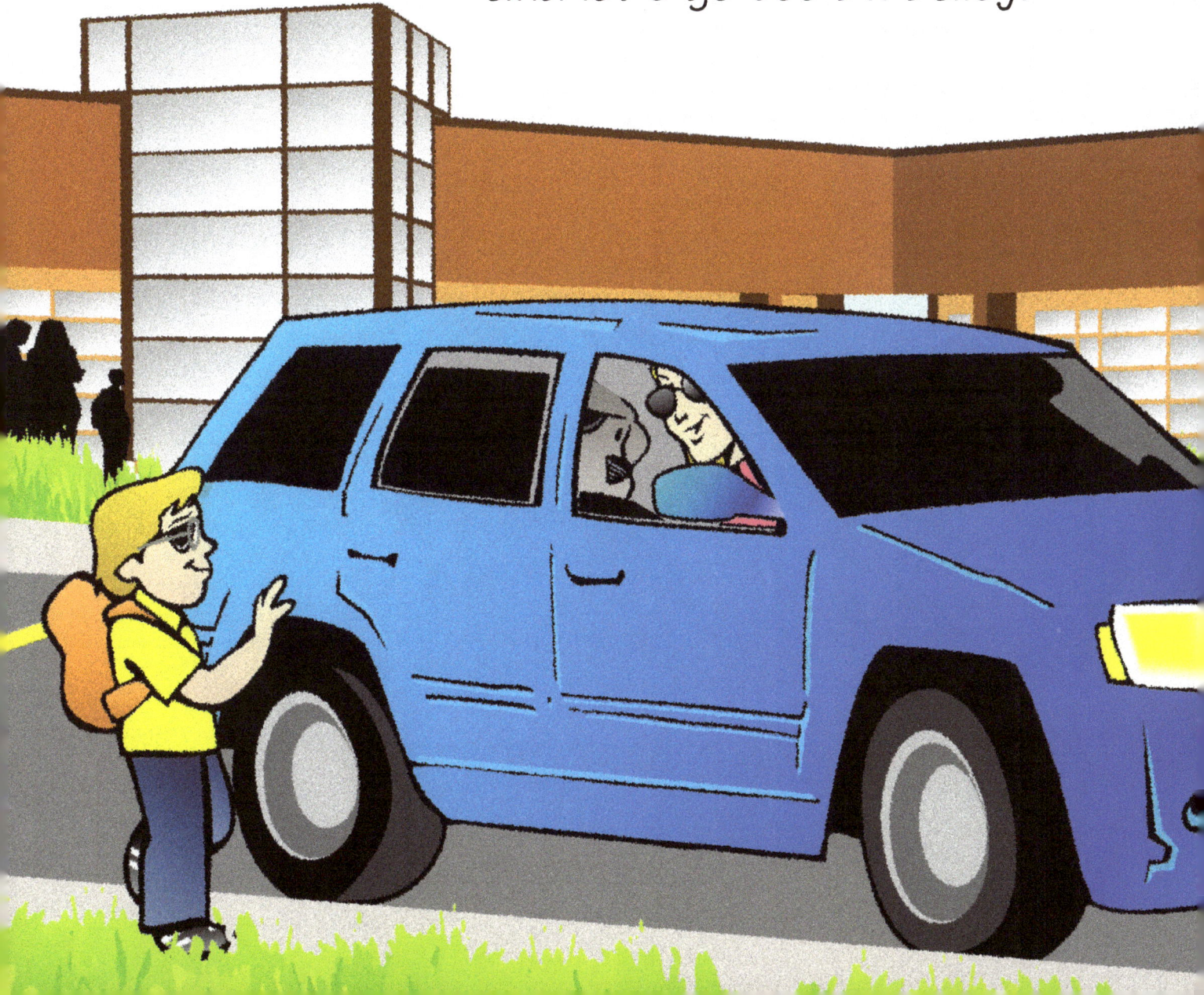

"Hello Preston. Buckle up and let's go see Dr. Daisy."

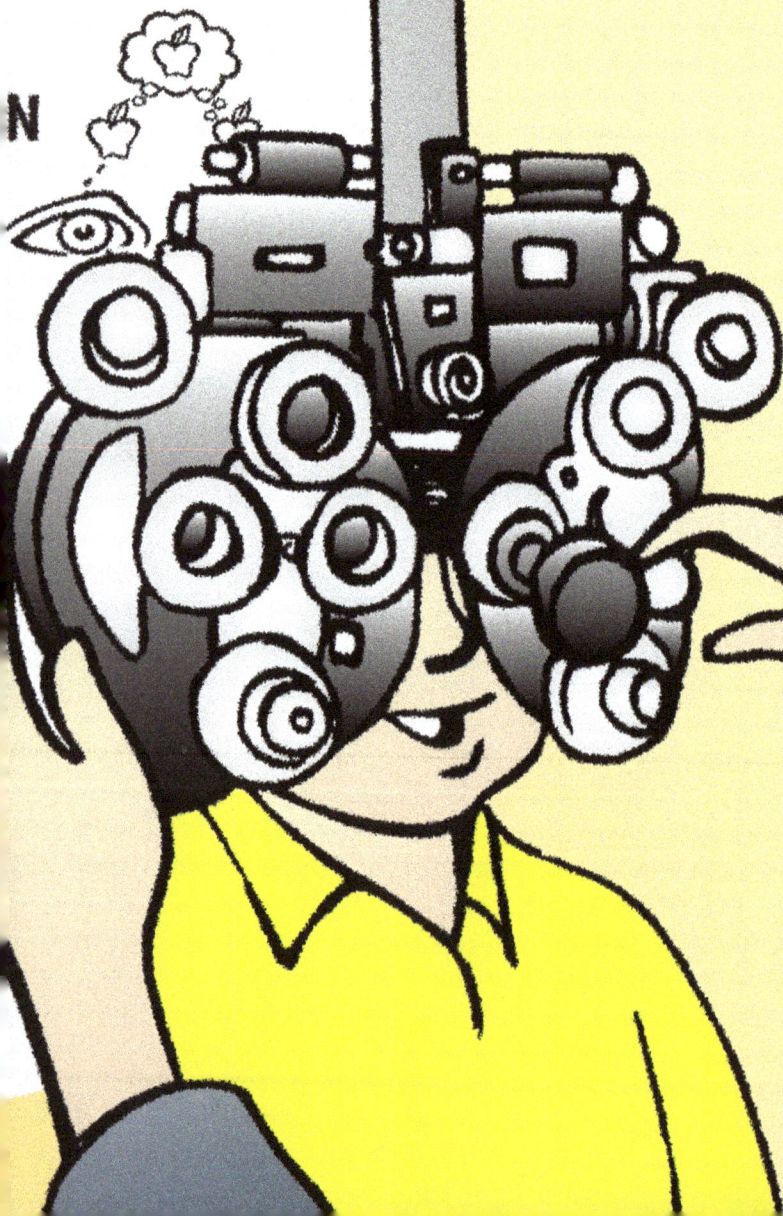

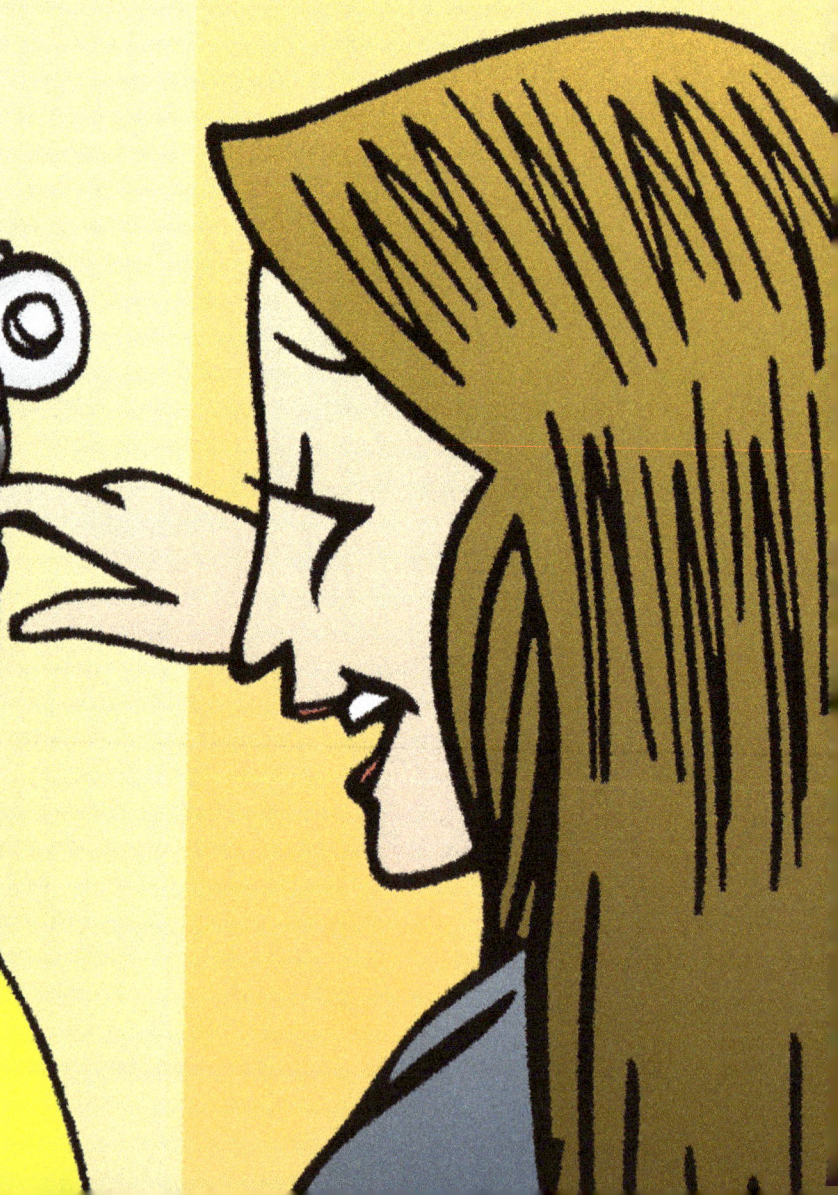

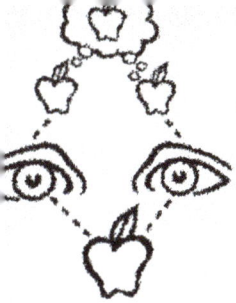

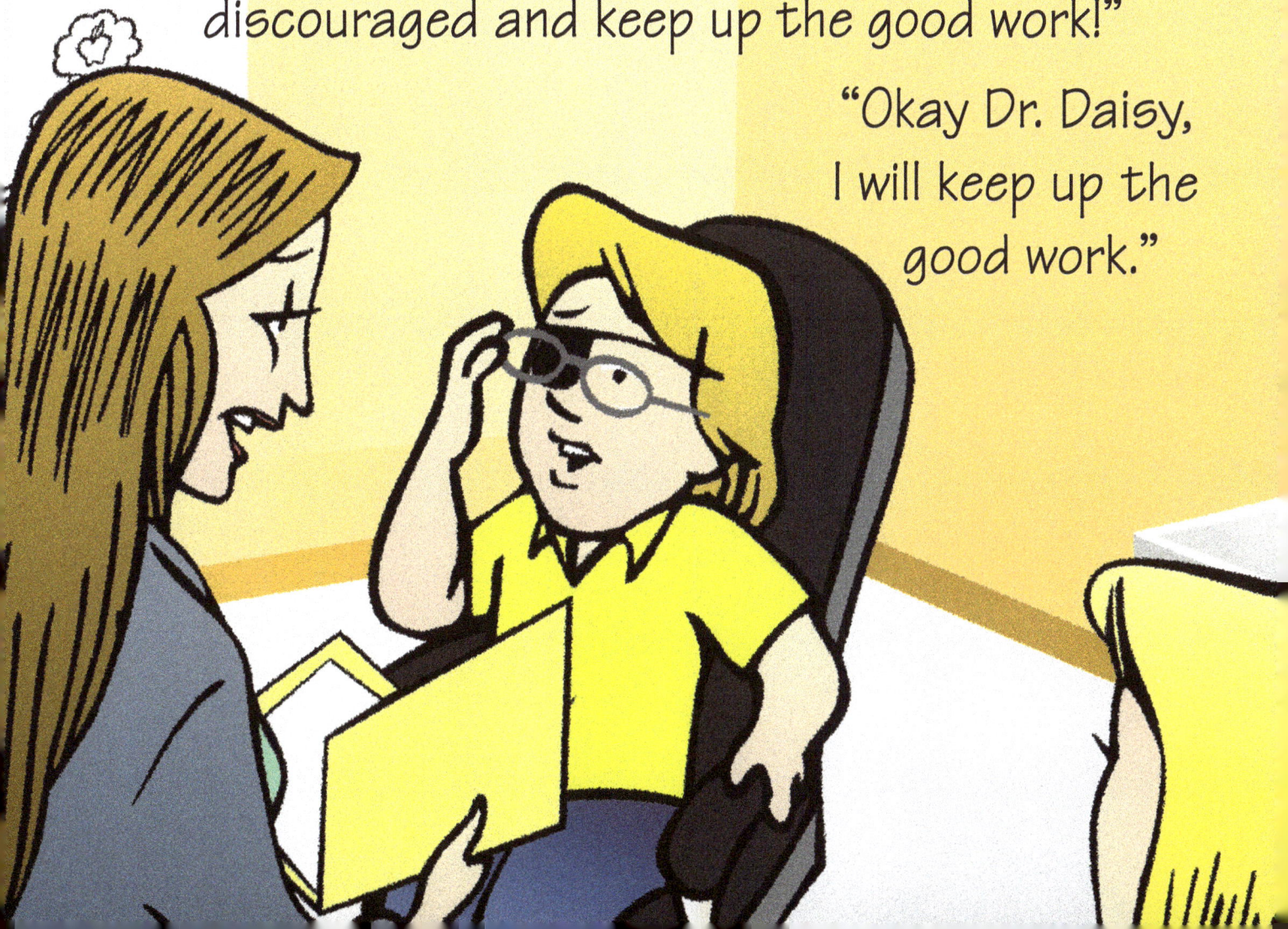

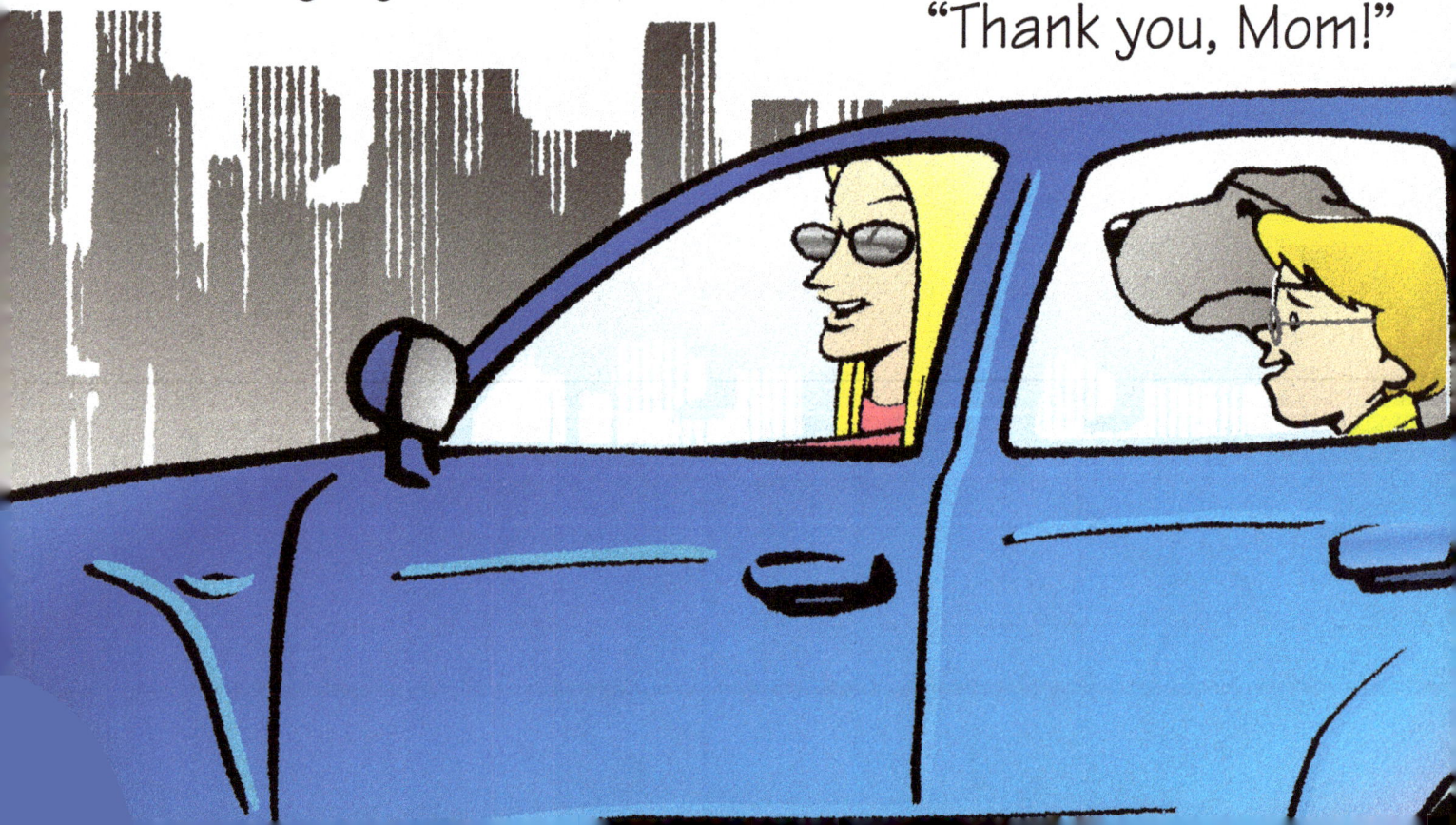

"Preston, I am very proud of you!"

"Mom, Dr. Daisy said I
didn't improve this time."

"Preston, if it wasn't for all your
efforts patching, you would not
be seeing as well as you are now.
Let's go get some ice cream."

"Thank you, Mom!"

"Preston, I cannot wait to hear about your next adventure in Patch Land."

"Here you go, Beau, and thank you for being my patch buddy and always going to Patch Land."

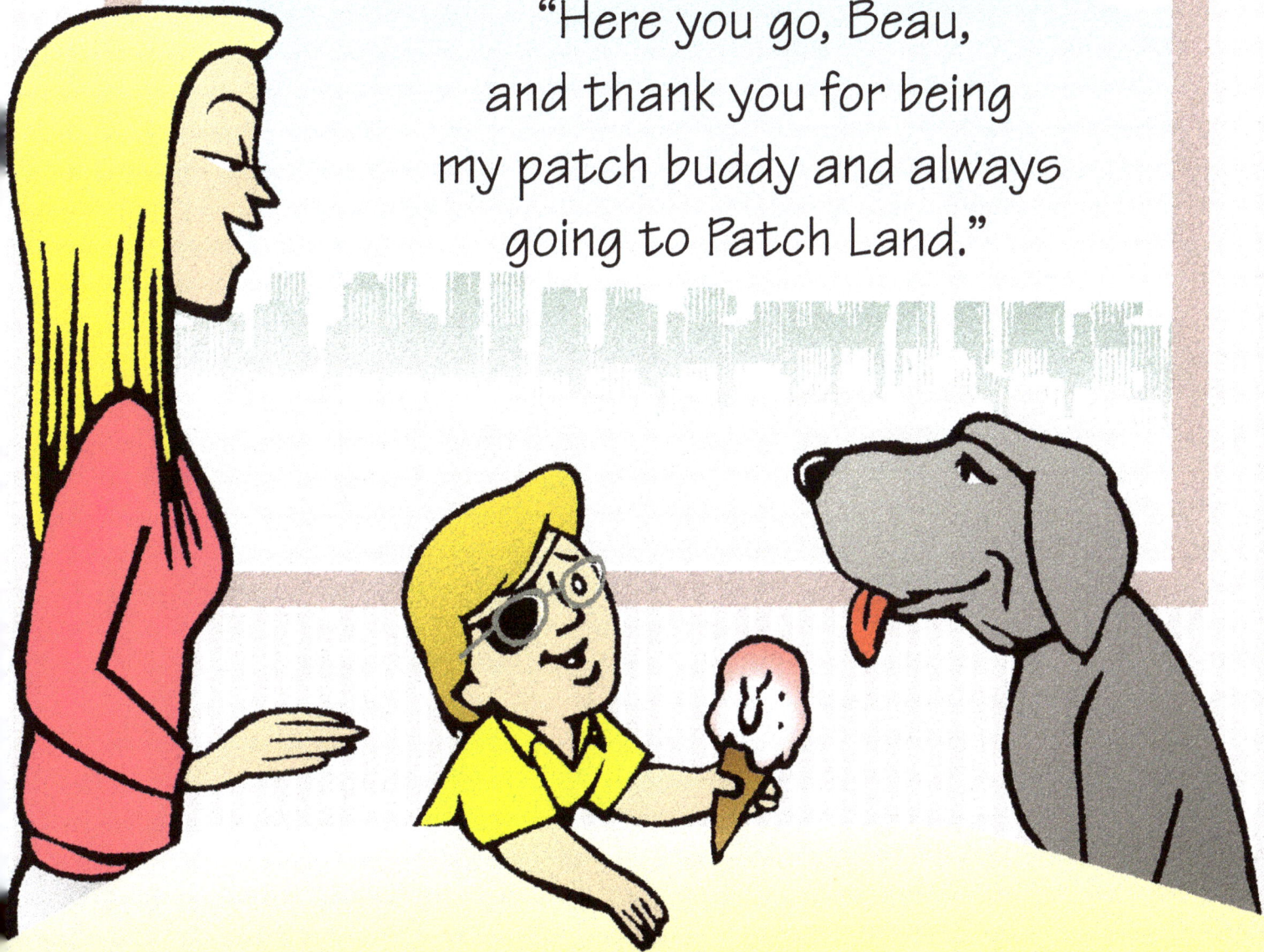

PATCH LAND ADVENTURES

BOOK THREE
WORK SHEET/COMPREHENSION

Name:

Date:

1) What kind of birthday party did Preston have?

2) What did Preston's cake and piñata look like?

3) During the birthday party, who broke the piñata?

4) Preston had a surprise visit for his birthday party, can you name who it was?

5) Do you remember the parrot's name?

6) During the treasure hunt, did they find the gold coins?

7) When the kids were in Patch Land, who scored the winning goal during the soccer game?

8) Preston went to the eye doctor after school, did his eye improve from his last visit?

9) What is the name of the illustrator?

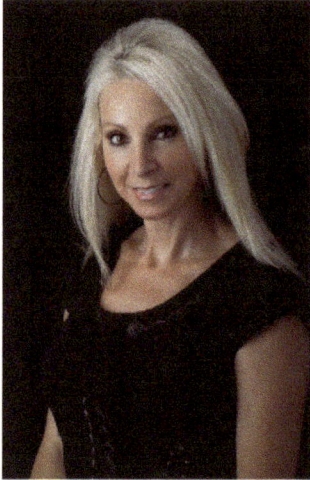

ABOUT THE AUTHOR

Author and speaker Carmen Swick lives in Colorado with her family where they enjoy many of the outdoor activities that the Centennial State has to offer. She volunteers with a non-profit organization, The Foundation Fighting Blindness, where she holds the position as President of the Denver Chapter. Outside of The Foundation Fighting Blindness she is the Chair for The Blind Taste of the Rockies, which is an annual fundraiser to raise awareness and search for a cure to blindness. In 2012 Carmen led the role of Chair for the Denver Vision Walk all the while attending schools for presentations/workshops and signings for the Patch Land Adventure series. Helping to find a cure for blindness isn't her only passion; she leads a team in the role of Captain in the Race for the Cure. She was the presenting children's book author for the 2014 Young Writers Conference for Jeffco Elementary Schools.

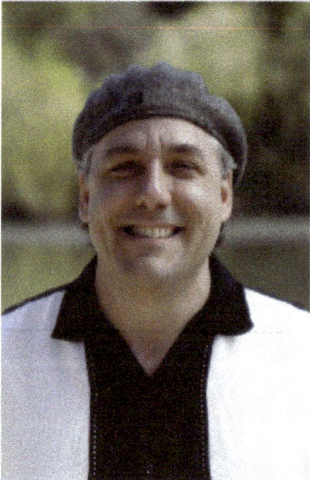

ABOUT THE ILLUSTRATOR

Joey Manfre is an illustrator and graphic artist with over twenty years of professional experience. Based in Northern California, he has worked on projects ranging from fancy wine packaging to funky tee shirts, but has a special fondness for illustrating books. For more information, check out his online portfolio at www.behance.net/joeyofdrawing.

Dedicated to Beau
January 8, 2002- June 12, 2015

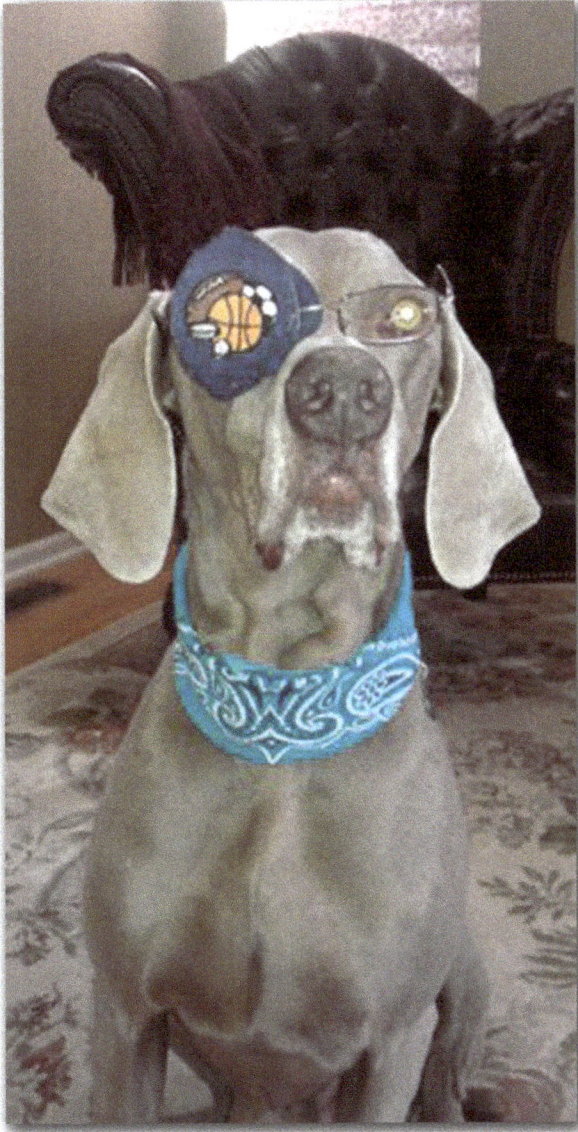

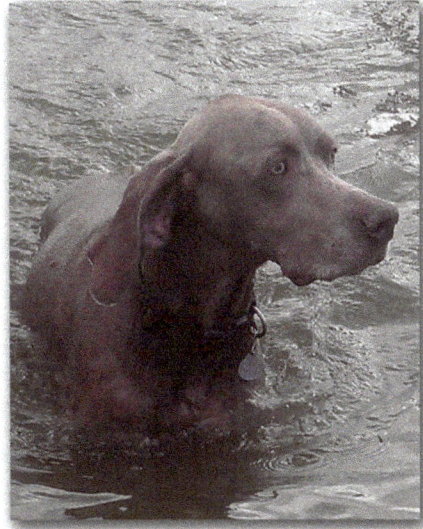

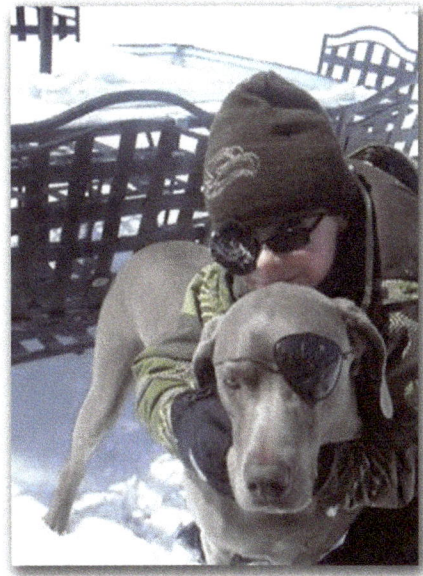

ABOUT AMBLYOPIA

Amblyopia is the leading cause of blindness in children. A condition in which a person's vision does not develop properly in early childhood because the eye and the brain are not working together correctly. Amblyopia, which usually affects only one eye, is also known as "lazy eye." A person with amblyopia experiences blurred vision in the affected eye. However, children often do not complain of blurred vision in the amblyopic eye because this seems normal to them. Early treatment is advisable, because if left untreated, this condition may lead to permanent vision problems.

For more information visit: Prevent Blindness at: http://www.preventblindness.org

Also Children's Eye Foundation: http://www.childrenseyefoundation.org

www.ingramcontent.com/pod-product-compliance
Lightning Source LLC
Chambersburg PA
CBHW051557030426
42334CB00034B/3470